Patient-Centered Medicine

Transforming the Clinical Method

Moira Stewart
Judith Belle Brown
W. Wayne Weston
Ian R. McWhinney
Carol L. McWilliam
Thomas R. Freeman

SAGE Publications
International Educational and Professional Publisher
Thousand Oaks   London   New Delhi

For information address:

 SAGE Publications, Inc.
2455 Teller Road
Thousand Oaks, California 91320

SAGE Publications Ltd.
6 Bonhill Street
London EC2A 4PU
United Kingdom

SAGE Publications India Pvt. Ltd.
M-32 Market
Greater Kailash I
New Delhi 110 048 India

Printed in the United States of America

Library of Congress Cataloging-in-Publication Data

Main entry under title:

Patient-centered medicine : transforming the clinical method /
    authors, Moira Stewart . . . [et al.].
        p.   cm.
    Includes bibliographical references and index.
    ISBN 0-8039-5688-6 (cloth). — ISBN 0-8039-5689-4 (pbk.)
    1. Medical personnel and patient.   2. Medicine—Philosophy.
I. Stewart, Moira.
    [DNLM: 1. Delivery of Health Care.   2. Physician-Patient
Relations.   3. Quality of Health Care.   4. Patient Participation.
5. Patient Satisfaction.   W 84 P298 1995]
R727.3.P364   1995
610—DC20
DNLM/DLC
for Library of Congress   94-43063

This book is printed on acid-free paper.

95   96   97   98   99   10   9   8   7   6   5   4   3   2

Production Editor: Diana E. Axelsen   Typesetter: Christina Hill

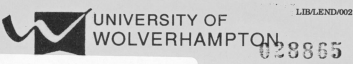

This book is dedicated to Joseph H. Levenstein, M.D.,
for his inspiration to the authors and his outstanding
contribution to the practice of medicine.

We are grateful to Dr. Levenstein for introducing us to the
Patient-Centered Clinical Method during his time as a
visiting professor in our Department in 1981–1982.

Contents

Foreword

The Department of Family Medicine of The University of Western Ontario has a long and proud record of defining the philosophy, science, principles, context, and process of Family Medicine. Their longtime internationally acclaimed leader, Ian McWhinney, systematically recruited and mentored a critical mass of gifted, industrious, and insightful scholars and clinicians who researched and executed these contributions. This book on the Patient-Centered Method, authored by Moira Stewart and several of those talented individuals, is one further contribution, this time to the enhancement of our understanding of a clinical method which is believed to be valid not only for Family Medicine but for all medicine. The latter statement is particularly significant in the current climate of health care reform and the need for a change of paradigm in medicine and medical education in response to societal needs.

It is in this vein that Ian McWhinney sets the stage in a chapter entitled "Why We Need a New Clinical Method." He argues cogently for the abandonment of the Cartesian mind/body split. Furthermore, he implies that we should abandon the concept of biopsychosocial components of illness, because we need to view all three components as intertwined and indivisible in our healing and management.

The body of the book relates to elaborating on the Patient-Centered Clinical Method—in chapters such as "Exploring Disease and Illness," "Understanding the Whole Person," and "Finding Common Ground"—as well as integrating into the model well-established principles of Family Medicine—in chapters such as "Incorporating Prevention and Health Promotion," and "Enhancing the Doctor-Patient Relationship," and in the discussion of appropriate usage of time and resources ("Being Realistic"). These chapters are rich with analysis, they review current literature, and they utilize examples of interactions to illustrate the many points that are made.

Inherent in the conceptualization of the Patient-Centered Method is the hope that this will more easily allow for "Teaching and Learning," a subject which is dealt with in the penultimate chapters of the book. Again this section provides a review of key learning methods. The assumption is made that learners already have a background in the biomedical world; now, what needs to be added is the undertaking of the human dimension of learning. This fact is underlined by the content of the very useful chapter on "Dealing With Common Difficulties in Learning and Teaching." All of the difficulties from teacher inexperience to self-awareness to the preoccupation with diagnosis and management arise from the reality that training in the biomedical method will have taken place first. A key assumption of the model, namely, "The Discomfort With Relinquishing Power to Patients" is dealt with in this section. This "difficulty," more than any other, epitomizes the changes required from the traditional value system that are needed if patients are to be regarded as responsible and responsive individuals capable of meeting challenges. "Listening" is an essential ingredient of the model and is in itself difficult for learners armed with the power that the biomedical model has given them. It should come as no surprise that the instructional method outlined for the patient-centered method is entitled the learner-centered method. It involves proceeding through the same conceptualization that has been applied to the Patient-Centered Clinical Method.

Finally, there is a review of the research on the limited activity that has been done to date of patient-centeredness and the methodology of the authors and others. Although it is accepted that this is just the beginning, we need to be reminded of McWhinney's earlier comment that the moral basis of the patient-centered method with its sharing of power should be enough to justify its introduction.

Moira Stewart and her coworkers are to be congratulated on putting together this book, which brings us up-to-date on the development of the patient-centered method. Yet much more needs to be done since the patient-centered method must be seen in the context of medical education and patient care and as a response to society's current health care expectations. To effect the patient-centered method in medical education requires a change in the medical school culture and value system and consequently the evaluation system itself. This book is the first landmark in this long journey and hopefully might spur many others in the years to come in the pursuit of a more caring and responsive patient and community-centered health care delivery system.

JOSEPH H. LEVENSTEIN, M.D.

Acknowledgments

This book represents more than 12 years of work by the authors. Such sustained effort occurs only in a supportive environment. We gratefully acknowledge Dr. Brian Hennen, Chair of the Department of Family Medicine, The University of Western Ontario; and Dr. Martin Bass, Director of the Centre for Studies in Family Medicine, for providing such an environment.

The ideas contained in this book evolved with the help of our patients, our students, and our colleagues both here in London and around the world.

The Canadian Library of Family Medicine (Lynn Dunikowski, Director, and staff) provided invaluable assistance with the reference list for this book.

We thank Rita Morgan for secretarial coordination of this project and Magda Valencia and Carol Leffley for secretarial support.

The research was conducted in the Thames Valley Family Practice Research Unit, which is supported by the Ministry of Health of Ontario as a Health System-Linked Research Unit. The ideas and conclusions contained in this book are those of the authors, and no endorsement by the ministry is intended or should be inferred.

Over the past 7 years, the authors have appreciated the encouragement of the Ontario Medical Association and the Committee on Medical Care and Practice, and the forum provided by the Ontario Medical Review in the column, *A Time to Talk, A Time to Listen.*

Introduction

MOIRA STEWART

W. WAYNE WESTON

Patients are dissatisfied. Physicians are confused and may no longer enjoy their work. Their training has not prepared them adequately for the everyday challenges in practice. After enduring the anxiety inherent in the transition from medical training to practice, the physician is faced with expectations that were never anticipated. There are competing demands on the doctor for his or her time, availability, and commitment. Confronted with complex patient problems and shrinking resources, the physician can be easily overwhelmed by the responsibilities of practicing medicine.

Why has this unsatisfactory situation arisen? In our view, the conventional models and methods of medicine and medical education have failed us, to some extent, in that they are incomplete and too narrow. The conventional biomedical approach ignores the person with the disease. To redress the balance, we suggest a revised model for medicine and medical education that includes the conventional biomedical approach but that also goes beyond it to include consideration of the patient as a person. We call this the "patient-centered model."

In this book, the patient-centered model of medicine is described and explained. A program of conceptual development, research, and education that has been underway for the past decade provides the material. Although the program took place in the context of family medicine, its messages are relevant, we believe, to all disciplines of medicine, to nursing, and to other health professions.

The patient-centered model of care presupposes a change in the mind-set of the clinician. The hierarchical notion of the professional being in charge and the patient being passive does not hold here. To be patient-centered, the practitioner must be able to empower the patient, to share the power in the relationship; this means renouncing control that traditionally has been in the hands of the professional. This is the moral imperative of patient-centered practice. In making this shift in values, the practitioner experiences the new direction the relationship can take when power is relinquished and shared.

In this book, we describe a patient-centered model of six interacting components. The first three interacting components encompass the process between patient and doctor. The second three components focus more on the context within which patient and doctor interact.

The first component of the patient-centered clinical model is the assessment of the two conceptualizations of ill health: disease and illness. In addition to assessing the disease process by history and physical examination, the physician actively seeks to enter into the patient's world to understand his or her unique experience of illness. Specifically, the doctor explores the patient's ideas about the illness, how the patient feels about being ill, what he or she expects from the physician, and how the illness affects the patient's functioning.

The second component is the integration of these concepts of disease and illness with an understanding of the whole person. This includes an awareness of the patient's position in the life cycle and the context in which he or she lives.

The mutual task of finding common ground between doctor and patient is the third component of the method and focuses on three key areas: (a) defining the problem, (b) establishing the goals of management, and (c) identifying the roles to be assumed by doctor and patient.

The fourth component highlights the importance of using each visit as an opportunity for prevention and health promotion.

The fifth component emphasizes that each contact with the patient should be used to build on the patient-physician relationship, including empathy, trust, caring, and healing.

The sixth component requires that, throughout the process, the physician be realistic about time, availability of resources, and amount of emotional and physical energy needed.

Societal and Professional Pressures for a New Model and Method

A remarkable number of changes in our society influence the patient-physician relationship. The Committee on Medical Care and Practice of the Ontario Medical Association (1992) has catalogued many of these societal changes and how they challenge the traditional practice of medicine (see Table I.1). Some of these changes may improve the interaction between patients and doctors (for example, emphasis on patient autonomy, interest in multiculturalism, and increased attention by the public on prevention and health education). All of these changes give patients power to become more involved in their own health care. But some of the changes may create new difficulties for doctors. For example, many doctors feel uncomfortable with the competing demands placed on them; they feel a conflict of interest between their commitment to their patients' welfare and the need to contain costs. The increasingly litigious environment and the increased liability of hospitals for doctors' care may lead to defensive approaches to practice. Doctors may feel limited by protocols and wary of what they say to patients.

Medicine is undergoing a radical transformation that demands fundamental changes in the way we conceptualize the role of physicians. These changes relate to major shifts in the fabric of society just mentioned. Many patients now demand a more egalitarian relationship with their physicians and expect to take a more active part in decisions about their health care. But many people, notably the elderly, still value the conventional model of the doctor who "always knows best."

Two manifestations of these challenges have been identified in the literature. First, communication problems between doctors and patients are relatively common; 50% of patients' complaints and 80% of

TABLE I.1 Medicine: The Changing Scene

Some of the changes affecting the patient-doctor relationship

— Rise of consumerism in medicine

— Shift of care from hospital to community

— Increased attention to prevention and patient education

— Changing status of women in society

— Emphasis on patient autonomy

— Doctor's role as trustee regarding disability benefits

— Increased awareness of physician's sexual abuse of patients

— Increased hospital liability for doctor's care

— Administrative containment of medical care costs

— Increasingly litigious environment

— Increased use of technology

— Social acceptance of physician-assisted suicide

— Multiculturalism

— Social concerns about woman assault and violence

— Holistic and alternative health movement

— Increased emphasis on informed consent

— Change in status of all professions in society—decline of role of medicine and expansion in role of other professionals

— Attacks on professional self-regulation

— The rise of a disabled culture of affirmative action and pride

SOURCE: Unpublished report, "Strategic goals: Report on the doctor-patient relationship and doctor-patient communication," prepared by the Ontario Medical Association Committee on Medical Care and Practice, Toronto, Ontario, Canada (December 1992).

social problems are not known to the physician (Stewart & Buck, 1977), and agreement on the need for follow-up between doctors and patients is also quite low (66.4%; Starfield et al., 1981). In addition, communication problems are serious in the intensity of patients' reactions of dissatisfaction; the majority of letters of complaint to health maintenance organizations (HMOs) (R. Frankel, personal communication, 1994) and complaints to disciplinary bodies are due to communication breakdown between the patient and the physician (College of Physicians and Surgeons of Ontario, 1988).

In the light of these findings about communication problems in the context of societal pressures, we agree with Stephens (1982) that "one of the paradoxes of our time is that the healing relationship seems most in jeopardy at a time when we need it most" (p. 38).

History of the Development
of the Patient-Centered Model

The Department of Family Medicine at The University of Western Ontario began its work on the patient-doctor relationship with the arrival of Dr. Ian McWhinney in 1968. His work elucidating the "real reason" the patient presented to the doctor (McWhinney, 1972) set the stage for explorations of breadth (all patient problems, whether physical, social, or psychological) and depth (the meaning of the patient's presentation). The research of Moira Stewart was guided by these interests and began to focus on the patient-physician relationship (Stewart & Buck, 1977; Stewart, McWhinney, & Buck, 1975, 1979).

In 1981-1982, Dr. Joseph Levenstein came from South Africa as a visiting professor of family medicine. He shared with us his patient-centered clinical method (Levenstein, 1984). During a typical day in his office in South Africa, seeing 30 patients with a variety of problems, he was challenged by a question from a medical student. She asked him how he knew what to do with each patient; his approach seemed so different from what she had seen in the hospital that she could not recognize any pattern to his technique. He explained that what he did was guided by his prior knowledge of each patient, by the frequency of different diseases in his community, and by the value he placed on continuity and comprehensiveness of care, prevention, and the doctor-patient relationship. He immediately sensed the student's bewilderment—his answer did not help her understand his method. He needed to be more specific if he was to help her practice in this way. Troubled by his inability to explain himself, he set about to find the answer. He began audiotaping his office consultations with patients and analyzing them. In the end, he reviewed about 1,000 audiotaped patient visits and concluded that his approach combined a traditional search for disease with an open-ended inquiry about whatever the patient wanted to discuss. He sorted the tapes into effective and ineffective interviews. He found that interviews in which he had elicited the patient's concerns and expectations about the visit went well; but if he missed the patient's cues to his or her "agenda," the interview was less effective. Here was something he could teach. Instead of exhorting his students to be more caring and leaving them confused and insulted, he could guide them to listen for patients' cues about their concerns, fears, and expectations and about why they presented themselves to the physician at that particular time. This feature of his approach was the basis for naming it the "patient-centered" method. This name harkens to the work of Rogers (1951) on client-centered counseling, Balint (1957) in person-centered medicine, Byrne and Long (1976) on doctor and patient-centered interviews, Newman and Young (1972) on total person approach to patient problems in nursing, and the "two-body practice" in occupational therapy (Mattingly & Fleming, 1994).

Levenstein refined his understanding of his method at Western and practiced teaching it to medical students and residents in family medicine with encouraging results. Residents understood what he meant and tried to change their behavior. Next, he taught the model to the faculty and collaborated in research to measure the impact of the method on patient care and teaching. The model had face validity for many of the faculty; some of us reacted with the feeling "Of course!" when we applied the model to our own work with patients and in our teaching. During the next year, the focus of the monthly faculty development sessions was on refining and elaborating the model. We have learned much since then by presenting the model to many groups of medical students, residents, graduate fellows, and community physicians and at numerous workshops for faculty across North America, Europe, Australia, and New Zealand.

Feedback from participants has been incorporated into the refinements of the model. As a result, the model was elaborated in several ways:

1. The conceptual distinction between disease (the pathological process) and illness (the unique experience of feeling unwell), first made by Fabrega (1978), was clarified.

2. Interviewing methods to discover the patient's experience were elucidated. "Patient's Ideas," "Expectations," "Feelings," and "Effects on Function" were incorporated into the model. It was important to understand patients within their social and developmental context.

3. An approach to finding common ground with patients was described.

4. We became aware of the work of Pendleton, Schofield, Tate, and Havelock (1984), who were defining independently a similar model of family practice. Their approach of defining their model as a set of tasks for the physician to perform in the consultation appealed to us, and we incorporated this idea into our own model. We refer to the elements of the model as "components," rather than as "tasks," to avoid the misconception that the model is a rigid, linear technique. The practice of medicine cannot be reduced to technique, but rather is embedded in a way of thinking about the tasks of medicine (White, 1988).

5. The model was expanded to include approaches to prevention, the doctor-patient relationship, and efficiency. It is important to note that the model was intended to be useful in understanding everyday encounters with patients; it was never intended to be a model focusing on psychotherapy or counseling, although it is useful also in understanding and helping patients with emotional problems.

Strengths and Limitations of Models

Epstein, Campbell, Cohen-Cole, McWhinney, and Smilkstein (1993) described, compared, and contrasted a number of approaches to patient-doctor communication, including the biopsychosocial model (Engel, 1977), the three-function model (Bird & Cohen-Cole, 1990), the family systems approach to patient care (Doherty & Baird, 1987; McDaniel, Campbell, & Seaburn, 1990), physician self-awareness (Balint, 1957), and the patient-centered model presented in this book. They concluded that "on a theoretical level, the complementarity of the approaches is more powerful than their difference" (Epstein et al., 1993, p. 386). In our view, the models are similar in their attempt to broaden the conventional medical approach to include psychosocial issues, the family, and the physician. The models differ in the level at which they work. Some are conceptual frameworks or models in the absence of a description of methods or behaviors for implementation. Others focus on practice behaviors within a less developed framework. Very few have been researched in any systematic way. One strength of the patient-centered model and the method we describe is that it includes both the theoretical framework or grounding and the strategies for implementation in practice, as well as a body of accompanying research.

Tresolini and Shugars (1994) described several models used by medical schools to integrate the biomedical and psychosocial domains. They used a qualitative methodology to examine 17 American and Canadian medical schools. They concluded:

> To fully enable students to learn an integrated approach to medical care, medical curricula should be patient-centered, integrated, developmental, and population-based throughout. . . . The evolving health care needs of the public have prompted a reconsideration of the biomedical model in medicine and the integration of psychosocial concerns in patient care. To prepare physicians who will be responsive to the current and future health care needs of the population, medical education must change accordingly. (pp. 235-236)

Models of patient-doctor communication in general, and the patient-centered model in particular, set out to make the implicit in patient care explicit. This is a necessary tool for teaching students and was certainly the motivation for Levenstein to begin developing his framework. Although models help clarify the basics in communication, they never completely capture what happens in reality. The tacit knowledge of the doctor and the patient are not captured in the models, which are, by definition, oversimplifications. Rudebeck (1992) pointed out that a model such as ours "sets norms for practical medicine by stressing one single aspect . . . [and does] not capture the very essence of practice" (pp. 67-68).

It should be added that, on the one hand, standardized classification and scoring procedures of quantitative research simplify even further the aspects of communication under consideration. Qualitative methodology, on the other hand, seeks to make the implicit, explicit.

Adopting a new conceptual framework and implementing new approaches in practice may sound very threatening to many medical practitioners. Are there risks as well as benefits in changing one's mind-set and methods to a patient-centered approach? Will patients be upset? Will office routine be slowed? Will the doctor be able to deal with all of the feelings expressed? We find that the benefits outweigh the potential risks.

For example, recent research in the United States, Canada, and elsewhere leads us to conclude that patient-centered visits are associated with such positive benefits as subsequent patient satisfaction and adherence (Stewart, 1984), reduction of concern (Bass et al., 1986; Headache Study Group of the University of Western Ontario, 1986; Henbest & Fehrsen, 1992; Henbest & Stewart, 1990), symptom reduction, and improved physiologic status (Greenfield, Kaplan, & Ware, 1988; Kaplan, Greenfield, & Ware, 1989b).

Research also has demonstrated that paying attention to the patient's illness does not result in less attention being paid to the traditional medical tasks of diagnosis and clinical management. Dutch and Canadian studies have shown no relationship between higher scores on patient-centered interviewing and lower scores on medical competence (Kraan & Crijnen, 1987; Stewart, Brown, & Weston, 1989).

Furthermore, research has indicated that patient-centered visits do not take longer than disease-centered visits. Two recent studies have shown that the length is virtually the same for visits we consider patient centered, compared with those scored at the other extreme (Greenfield et al., 1988; Stewart et al., 1989).

Another insight from research is that physicians who have learned the patient-centered method are flexible in their approach to individual patients. Physicians who have, on average, high patient-centered scores show a wide range in scores, implying a flexibility in practice (Stewart et al., 1989).

Finally, research has pointed out the challenges in teaching and learning the patient-centered approach. On the one hand, many of the methods we teach can be implemented by residents and practicing physicians during 6 to 12 weeks (e.g., considering patient's ideas and feelings; Stewart et al., 1989). On the other hand, students and physicians often have more difficulty with other aspects of the model (e.g., finding common ground). At first, they use the method as an add-on to the conventional clinical method and, when they are rushed, tired, or feeling threatened, they revert to a focus on disease. It takes considerable experience with the patient-centered model before it becomes second nature. Teachers need to keep in mind this natural history of learning the method and not become impatient or overly critical of students who have trouble integrating the method or who backslide under pressure.

Overview

This book is divided into three parts. Part One, describing the conceptual framework, begins with a historic perspective written by Ian R. McWhinney. Chapter 2 is a concise description of the six interacting components of the patient-centered model. Chapters 3 to 8 elaborate Components 1 to 6, respectively.

The clinical reader will notice the cases illustrating each of the six components of the patient-centered approach in Chapters 3 to 8. Readers most interested in the application of patient-centeredness in everyday practice might enjoy reading the cases first. Taken together, the cases represent a typical series of patients in the practice of a busy doctor.

Part Two, on teaching and learning, contains five chapters that move from the context of medical education (Chapter 9) to challenges and general solutions (Chapter 10). Chapter 11 contains details on teaching strategies and objectives, as well as a section drawing parallels between learner-centered teaching and patient-centered practice. Chapter 12 contains tips for teaching patient-centered medicine. Chapter 13 describes a particular teaching tool—the patient-centered case presentation.

Part Three, on research, combines reviews of relevant literature with results from recent studies conducted by the authors. Qualitative and quantitative methodologies are represented. Chapter 14 contains a formal review of quantitative studies correlating communication with patient health outcomes, demonstrating the efficacy of patient-centered components. Chapter 15 briefly describes a variety of measures available to the researcher wishing to embark on a quantitative study of communication in general and patient-centered communication in particular. Chapter 16 presents key findings from the interpretive tradition of research and draws parallels between the patient-centered clinical method and qualitative inquiry. The final chapter combines qualitative and quantitative findings regarding the evolution of patient-doctor relationships over time. The conclusion looks to the future and, taking into account the steps already taken, explores some possible fresh visions of concepts, teaching, and research on medical practice.

1

Why We Need a
New Clinical Method

IAN R. McWHINNEY

Medicine needs a new clinical method because, for all its great successes, our present method is failing to meet the needs of the late 20th century. Our diagnostic and therapeutic method, the structure of our profession, and the structure of the health care system are products of the Enlightenment, so it is not surprising that they should be in trouble at a time when the ideas of the Enlightenment themselves are exposing their weaknesses. There is irony here, for the new demands on our clinical method arise, to some extent, from the successes and failures of the Enlightenment project. Thus, as always, medicine proves to be a child of its time. These contentions require justification. First, however, it is necessary to trace the connections between clinical method and the ideas that have formed the modern world.

The Enlightenment

In the 16th and 17th centuries, Western Europeans experienced a change in worldview of momentous proportions. The cosmology of Copernicus, the discovery of new lands in the East and West, the settlement and exploitation of the New World, and the Protestant revolt against the Roman church all played their part in the rapid collapse of the medieval world order. It was out of this great ferment of ideas that modern science was born. A. N. Whitehead (1975) de-

1

scribed this new way of thinking as a coming together of an interest in detailed facts and a devotion to abstraction and generalization. All great civilizations have had their abstract thinkers, and all have had their practical people devoted to the detailed performance of their arts; it was the union of these interests in individuals that made European science unique.

Early European science was not without some precedents, however. Indeed, Whitehead described the Middle Ages as "one long training of the intellect of Western Europe in the sense of order . . . an epoch of orderly thought, rationalist through and through" (Whitehead, 1975, p. 23). This sense of the natural and moral order was essential to the development of science because, without a belief in the order of nature, it would have been fruitless to search for natural laws. The greatest contribution of the medieval world to the formation of the scientific movement was "the belief that every detailed occurrence can be correlated with its antecedents in a perfectly definite manner exemplifying general principles" (Whitehead, 1975, p. 24).

Science requires both this instinctive faith in rationality and an interest in the simple occurrences of life for their own sake. This interest in practical matters was already discernable in 6th-century Western Europe, where the early Benedictines lived lives that were both spiritual and practical. According to Whitehead (1975), the alliance of science with technology, by which learning is kept in contact with irreducible and stubborn facts, owes much to the practical bent of the early Benedictines. An echo of this is seen in John Ruskin's (1981) description of the Gothic mind as having a love of natural objects for their own sake. These Western European workers, with their delight in the representation of facts, built and adorned the great Gothic cathedrals of the Middle Ages.

Even though science and the medieval church shared this faith in reason and in the orderliness of nature, they soon came into conflict over the "facts." Galileo was interested in how things happen; his adversaries were interested in why things happen, and their metaphysical beliefs provided them with the answer. In the light of their a priori assumptions, their case was eminently reasonable but ignored what William James called "the irreducible and stubborn facts" (Whitehead, 1975, p. 13). This new interest in the world of facts was stimulated by epoch-making inventions such as the mechanical clock, the telescope, the ship's compass, and the printing press, that, together with the generalizations behind the facts, led to the great era of scientific creativity with which we are familiar. Whitehead called the 1600s the century of genius and asserted that we have lived ever since on the accumulated capital of its ideas. It was a century that contained the two towering figures of early modern science: Galileo and Newton. Also in the 16th century, the agenda of the Enlightenment was written by three men: Francis Bacon, René Descartes, and John Locke. Bacon urged humankind to dominate and control nature, thus lightening the miseries of existence. In *Advancement of Learning*, he provided, as his agenda for medical science, a revival of the Hippocratic method of recording case descriptions, with their course toward recovery or death; and the study of the pathological changes in organs—the "footsteps of disease"—with a comparison between these and the manifestations of illness during life (Faber, 1923, pp. 5-6). Clinical medicine at this time was dominated by a theory, not grounded in bedside observation. The new scientific ideas recently had been applied to medicine by such men as Vesalius and Harvey, but their discoveries had been in anatomy and physiology, not in pathology and clinical science.

Thomas Sydenham

In the intellectual climate of the 1600s arose the first modern physician to use systematic bedside observation: Thomas Sydenham. Sydenham described the symptoms and course of disease, setting aside all speculative hypotheses based on unsupported theories. He classified diseases into categories—a novel idea at the time—believing that they could be classified by description in the same way as botanical specimens. Finally, he sought a remedy for each "species" of disease, exemplified by the newly introduced Peruvian bark (quinine). His great innovation, however, was to correlate his disease categories with their course and outcome, thus giving them predictive value. His method bore fruit in the distinction, for the first time, of syndromes such as acute gout and chorea. Sydenham was a close friend of John Locke, who took a great interest in Sydenham's observations, sometimes accompanying him on visits to patients. Locke, also a physician, was one of the great figures of the Enlightenment—the father of empiricism and the philosopher who laid the groundwork for those features of the modern world: individualism, the concept of natural rights, and the dominance of reason torn from its metaphysical roots. The friendship between Locke and Sydenham is an interesting example of the connection between medicine and the dominant ideas of the time. Thomas Jefferson considered Bacon, Locke, and Newton to be the three greatest men of all time (Borgmann, 1992, p. 25).

If Bacon set the agenda for science, Descartes provided the method: the separation of mind and matter, with value residing only in mind; the separation of subject and object; and the reduction of complex phenomena to their simplest components.

From Sydenham to Laennec

After Sydenham, the work of classifying diseases was taken up by others, notably Sauvages of Montpellier, a physician and botanist who sought to group diseases into classes, orders, and genera in the same way that biologists classified plants and animals. Biology and medicine were at this time predominantly descriptive sciences. Sauvages was a strong influence on Carl von Linné, the Swedish physician and botanist responsible for the Linnaean system of botanical classification—another instance of the connection between medicine and the ideas of the Enlightenment. The groupings of Sydenham's successors were of little practical value, however, because they were not correlated with the course and outcome of disease and represented only random combinations of symptoms with no basis in the natural order.

Sydenham died in 1689, and for the next 100 years no system for classifying diseases proved to be of lasting value. The next great step, and the one that laid the foundations for the modern clinical method, was taken by the French clinician-pathologists in the years after the French Revolution. The political turmoil engendered by Enlightenment ideas was associated with a further application of these ideas to medicine. The method was described by Laennec, the greatest genius of the French school:

> The constant goal of my studies and research has been the solution of the following three problems:
> 1. To describe disease in the cadaver according to the altered states of the organs.
> 2. To recognize in the living body definite physical signs, as much as possible independent of the symptoms . . .

3. To fight the disease by means which experience has shown to be effective: . . . to place, through the process of diagnosis, internal organic lesions on the same basis as surgical disease. (Faber, 1923, p. 35)

For the first time, clinicians examined their patients by using new instruments such as the Laennec stethoscope. They then linked together two sets of data: (a) signs and symptoms from the clinical inquiry and (b) the descriptive data of morbid anatomy. At last, medicine had a classification system based on the natural order of things: the correlation between symptoms, signs, and the appearance of the organs and tissues after death. The system proved to have great predictive value. It was further vindicated when Pasteur and Koch showed that some of these entities had specific causal agents. The clinical method based on this system developed gradually during the 19th century, until by the 1870s it had taken the form familiar to us today.

As is always the case, this development in clinical method was associated with a change in the perception of disease. Since classical times, Western medicine has used two explanatory models of illness (Crookshank, 1926; Dubos, 1980). According to the *ontological model,* a disease is an entity located in the body and conceptually separable from the sick person. According to the *physiological* or *ecological model,* disease results from an imbalance within the organism and between organism and environment: Individual diseases have no real existence, the names being simply clusters of observations used by physicians as a guide to prognosis and therapy. According to the latter view, it becomes difficult to separate the disease from the person and the person from the environment.

Each model is identified with a clinical method: the ontological with a conventional method, and the physiological with a natural method. Crookshank (1926), who introduced these terms, also observed that the best physicians in all ages used a balance of the two methods. The patient-centered clinical method can be seen as the restoration of balance to a clinical method that has gone too far in the ontological direction.

The success of the new clinical method in the late 1800s soon resulted in a dominance of the ontological model, a dominance it has retained ever since. Whereas in former times the word *diagnosis* often meant the diagnosis of a patient, the aim of diagnosis now was to identify the disease. Disease was located in the body. As in all taxonomies, the disease categories were abstractions that, in the interest of generalization, left out many features of illness, including the subjective experience of the patient. Mental and physical diseases were classified separately, except for the group known as "psychosomatic diseases." Psychotherapy became distinguished from somatic therapy. In accordance with the dictates of reason and objectivity, the physician was viewed as a detached and impassive observer.

With its predictive and inferential power, the new clinical method was highly successful. Indeed, the application of new technologies to medicine depended on it. It had other strengths too: It gave the clinician a clear injunction to "identify the patient's disease or rule out organic pathology"; it broke down a complex process into a series of easily remembered steps; and it provided canons of verification. The pathologist was able to tell the clinician whether he or she was right or wrong.

So successful was the method that its weaknesses became apparent only much later, as its abstractions became further and further removed from the experience of the patient. True to its origins in the age of reason, the method was analytical and impersonal. Feelings and the life experience of the patient did not figure in the process. The meaning of the illness was established on one level only—that of physical pathology. In keeping with the ontological model of disease, the focus was on diagnosis, with much less attention to the detailed care of the patient. In keeping also with its Cartesian origins, it divided mental from physical disorder, bringing the two together in such dubious terms as "functional illness," "psychosomatic disease," and "neurotic overlay." This dichotomy between the mental and the physical was represented eventually in the organization of the profession. Neurology and internal medicine became separated from psychiatry, pediatrics from child psychiatry, and geriatrics from psychogeriatrics. It also was reflected in medical institutions: different wards, units, and hospitals for mental and physical diseases.

The central idea on which our clinical method was based came into being at a time when Enlightenment ideas had become the dominant worldview of the West. The human being had become the measure of all things, metaphysics was devalued, tradition was weakened, progress was proclaimed, and knowledge was put to practical use for the benefit of humankind. Reason was enthroned, but it was a reason defined as formal logic, divorced from human experience. The fruits borne by these ideas in our own time include our clinical method and all of the benefits and problems of modern medicine. Some of the other fruits have a particular bearing on the critique of clinical method: moral relativism, the modern paradigm of knowledge, and the severance of our culture from its traditions. Knowledge in our own time has become instrumental, defined, and valued as a means to produce certain ends. Our universities and medical schools are dominated by this paradigm. Knowledge that matters is impersonal, public, productive, and empirically verifiable. Knowledge that is personal, tacit, experiential, or intuitive is hardly recognized as knowledge.

One view of the origins of the modern paradigm of knowledge is that it arose quite abruptly from the medieval world in the 17th century. According to Stephen Toulmin (1992), this view misses a short but important period in the history of Western Europe: the flowering of a humanistic culture in the 16th century. Whereas 17th-century thinkers aimed to frame their questions in terms that rendered them independent of context, those of the previous century balanced their theoretical inquiries with discussion of concrete practical issues as they arise in questions of medical diagnosis, legal liability, or moral responsibility: "They regarded human affairs in a clear-eyed nonjudgmental light that led to honest practical doubt about the value of 'theory' for human experience—whether in theology, natural philosophy, metaphysics, or ethics" (Toulmin, 1992, p. 25). They were interested in practical knowledge, the oral, the particular, the local, and the timely: the knowledge that comes from the application of reason to individual cases. The representative figures in this period were Eramus, Montaigne, and Shakespeare. From the 17th century onward, this knowledge was devalued in favor of the written, the general, the universal, and the timeless. Knowledge became decontextualized. This reflected

a historical shift from practical philosophy, whose issues arose out of clinical medicine, juridical procedure, and moral case analysis . . . to a theoretical conception of philosophy. . . . Thus, from 1630 on, the focus of philosophical inquiries has ignored the particular, concrete, timely, and local details of every day human affairs: instead it has shifted to a higher, stratospheric place on which nature and ethics conform to abstract, timeless, general, and universal theories. (Toulmin, 1992, pp. 34-35)

Clinical medicine, it seems, took a long time to fall under the domination of this paradigm of knowledge. Although the new clinical method was concerned with abstractions, until our own century the individual case or series of cases remained the focus of attention for study and for teaching. Our abstractions have been low level—not far removed from experience of patients. In more recent times, however, the development of our clinical method can be seen as moving toward increasing levels of abstraction and an increasing distance from the experience of illness. Given the identification of medicine with the modern university, it could hardly escape becoming "decontextualized." The fact that a ward round now can be done round the charts rather than round the beds is an indication of how far we have gone.

The Worm in the Apple

The shortcomings of the new clinical method were a reflection of the failures of the whole Enlightenment project. Even in the 17th and 18th centuries, some prophetic spirits already were seeing a worm in the Enlightenment apple. Swift and Blake, in Britain, and Pascal, in France, were quick to tell those few who would listen that a price was to be paid for its benefits. Later came the Romantic revolt against the Enlightenment, with Wordsworth and Coleridge as leading figures in the English-speaking tradition. Their message was a simple one. When we make abstractions, something dies. When cold reason drives out imagination, what dies is the spirit. In his autobiographical poem "The Prelude," Wordsworth (1988) addressed these lines to his friend Coleridge:

> No officious slave
> Art thou of that false secondary power
> By which we multiply distinctions, then
> Deem that our puny boundaries are things
> That we perceive and not that we have made. (p. 85, lines 15 to 19)

Our world now is dominated by these "puny boundaries" between mind and body, biological and psychosocial, fact and value, subject and object, observer and observed. But can we agree with Wordsworth that they are indeed puny or that making abstractions is a false and secondary power? Abstractions are certainly not false in the sense of untrue. An abstraction can reveal to us truths about nature that unfold over the years. In another sense, however, abstractions are false; they are only partial truths. No abstraction can represent fully the experience from which it abstracts. If it did, it would not be an abstraction and would lose its generalizing power.

Few would disagree with Wordsworth that abstraction is a secondary power. The primary power, both in terms of human development and of human value, is our capacity for spontaneous, prereflective, intuitive response to experience. It is a power exemplified best by young children and by people in preliterate cultures. Owen Barfield (1957) called it "participating consciousness": the direct experience of nature without the intervention of schemata and abstractions and without the separation of subject and object. In our culture, as we grow older, this power weakens as we experience the world increasingly through the lens of our internalized abstractions.

Atrophy of participating consciousness leads to a kind of spiritual death. As Wordsworth expressed it in his poem "The Tables Turned":

> *Our meddling intellect*
> *Misshapes the beauteous forms of things:*
> *We murder to dissect.* (lines 26-28)

It is the same disenchantment felt by Mark Twain, who found, when he had gained the intellectual mastery needed to pilot the Mississippi, that the river had lost its beauty for him (Pirsig, 1974, p. 77).

The problem was referred to by Whitehead (1975) as the fallacy of misplaced concreteness, of mistaking our abstractions for reality; to Alfred Korzybski, it was mistaking the map for the territory; and to James (1958), it was eating the menu instead of the meal. In a famous passage in *The Varieties of Religious Experience*, William James (1958) wrote:

> The first thing the intellect does with an object is to class it along with something else. But any object that is infinitely important to us . . . feels to us also as if it must be sui generis and unique. Probably a crab would be filled with a sense of personal outrage if it could hear us class it . . . as a crustacean, and thus dispose of it. "I am no such thing," it would say; "I am MYSELF, MYSELF alone." (p. 26)

This is not simply a question of either/or. There are gains as well as losses in abstraction. The secondary power of abstraction is essential to our well-being and survival. Even preliterate people have their abstractions. Hunter-gathers, for example, have to distinguish between edible and poisonous plants. The problem comes when the secondary power overwhelms the first and when our abstractions impoverish our experience. The purpose of philosophy, said Whitehead (1975), is to criticize our abstractions, lest we become their prisoners.

The Tasks of Medicine

Our first task is to recapture the capacity to respond to our patients prereflectively and spontaneously. As Kay Toombs (1992) put it, a patient wants to be recognized, appreciated, and understood. This means responding to a patient's suffering. One of medicine's perennial moral problems—and one almost totally ignored by modern bioethics—is a failure to respond to suffering. Responding to suffering is not a question of categories. As Arthur Frank (1991) said in his book *At the Will of the Body:* "Caring has nothing to do with categories; it shows the person that her life is valued because it recognizes what makes her experience particular" (p. 48). We respond to suffering— and to other expressions of the human condition—not by analyzing them and not only by words, for some of the things we want to express cannot be expressed by words alone, but by a movement of our whole being. Perhaps it is best described as a dance. Martha Graham is said to have responded to someone who asked the meaning of a dance: "If I could tell you, I wouldn't need to dance it." Let me give as an example an experience described by Oscar Wilde (1915). Wilde had been imprisoned for an offense related to his homosexuality. He was impoverished, humiliated, separated from his children, declared bankrupt, and deserted by most of his friends. While in Reading Gaol, he wrote:

> Where there is sorrow there is holy ground. Some day people will realize what that means. They will know nothing of life till they do. . . . When I was brought down from my prison to the Court of Bankruptcy, between two policemen, [Robert Ross] waited in the long dreary corridor that, before the whole crowd, whom an action so sweet and simple hushed

into silence, he might gravely raise his hat to me, as, handcuffed and with bowed head, I passed him by. . . . When wisdom has been profitless to me, philosophy barren, and the proverbs and phrases of those who have sought to give me consolation as dust and ashes in my mouth, the memory of that little, lovely, silent act of love has unsealed for me the wells of pity: made the desert blossom like a rose, and brought me out of the bitterness of lonely exile into harmony with the wounded, broken, and great heart of the world. (pp. 25-26)

Robert Ross's act of recognition was simply being present for his friend and performing the sign of recognition that was appropriate for the time: raising his hat. It was what the French call an *acte de présence.*

If our clinical method does not have this recognition as its overriding theme, transcending all dualisms and all categories, it will fail at its deepest level. This is not just the beginning; it is the beginning, the middle, and the end. It means that although we can use our maps, we must never lose sight of the territory. In the clinical encounter, it may find expression in a hundred different ways: listening with undivided attention to the patient's story, sitting at the bedside, attending to the smallest need, being present at a critical time, asking a question that releases pent-up feelings. These are symbolic acts. I think we almost have forgotten that our every act is symbolic. It is through transcendent symbols that we express our deepest feelings.

This recognition provides the context for an understanding of what the illness means for the patient and what the patient expects from the doctor. To be patient-centered, every clinical encounter should result in some answers to these questions: What is the patient's understanding of the illness? What does the patient believe caused it? What are his or her expectations of the doctor? What are his or her feelings? What are his or her fears? Toombs (1992) said that fears are nearly always specific. Will I lose the use of my legs? Will I be able to get to the toilet in time? "No neurologist," said Toombs, a sufferer for 15 years from multiple sclerosis, "has ever asked me if I am afraid." Finally, we should have a feeling for the impact of the illness on the patient's life: the limitations, disabilities, effect on relationships, work, interests, hopes, and aspirations. The understanding attained by using the patient-centered method should lead naturally to an attempt to attain common ground, a mutual understanding of the nature of the illness. But to see the patient-centered method only in terms of the doctor's understanding of the patient is to take too limited a view. Our clinical method should be a process in which meanings are shared. The meaning of an illness in terms of its physical pathology (the clinical diagnosis), for example, will be conveyed from doctor to patient and clarified by dialogue until there is a shared understanding of the meaning in all of its ramifications. The process is circular, not linear, and the shared understanding often is different from the initial understanding of both doctor and patient.

Boundaries

Now we come to the secondary power. Much of the power of our clinical method comes from its capacity to classify the patient's illness very precisely. There are four good reasons for classifying a patient's illness.

First, it can give us great predictive power, an answer to that ever-present question: What is going to happen to me? Second, it can point us to the effective remedy for the disease. If we look at the history of some of our disease categories, we find that their emergence coincides with that of an effective remedy. When I started in practice, there was no such disease category as polymyalgia rheumatica. The first patient I saw with this illness was unclassifiable. A consultant suggested I try prednisone, and the result, of course, was dramatic. During the next few years, I followed in the literature the emergence of this new disease category.

Third, classification gives us a common vocabulary and language so that we can discuss our experience with colleagues, both in person and in the literature. Fourth, it names the patient's illness. Giving the illness a name can have great symbolic significance for a patient (Wood, 1991). It may say, "You are not alone. Your illness is not some vague hidden menace, but a familiar thing." Note, however, that to give this assurance, the named category does not need to have powers of prediction and causal inference. Some common categories, such as irritable colon syndrome, are little more than restatements of the patient's symptoms. Sometimes they are more important for stating what the patient does *not* have. For example, irritable colon syndrome says "You do not have cancer."

Note also that effective classification and treatment may proceed without our knowing the "cause" of the disease. We still do not know the cause of polymyalgia rheumatica, but we can treat it effectively. Causal thinking is deeply entrenched in our culture. No sooner has a phenomenon been described than the question of its cause begins to be asked, and cause usually is viewed as a one-way relationship between a single agent and a single effect on a passive organism or object. People have always sought explanations for their illnesses and misfortunes, but there is a difference between an explanation and an attribution of cause. The *explanation* of an illness, as of an ecological change, may be more in the nature of a disturbance of balance or harmony than the *attribution* of an effect to a specific agent. Many of the illnesses we encounter cannot be attributed to specific causal agents. Even when they can, the agent is only one part of a complex web of relationships. We seem to be obsessed by causal thinking, particularly by the question that can only arise in a dualistic culture: Is it physical or mental?

This is one reason why we often fail with illnesses such as chronic fatigue. We search for physical causes. Finding none, we either assume that we have solved the problem by excluding "disease" or that the illness is psychological. No wonder our patients get angry and form themselves into groups of activists. Papers are published describing the search for a causal agent, often assuming that the cause is a single external agent, rather than a number of environmental agents triggering a process that is already a potential of the organism.

Consider now how a different way of thinking might help the patient. First would come the recognition of the patient's sufferings and an understanding of the personal meaning of the illness. Second would come the diagnostic search, excluding other categories of disease associated with fatigue, especially those readily remediable. Third would come the naming of the illness and the explanation, which would turn the patient's attention from thinking about cause to thinking about healing. We know that the human organism has a great capacity for healing; our therapy must be directed toward assisting nature in this process. This will require attention to diet, rest, exercise, and the environment. Because support is crucial, we will need to help the patient's family and colleagues provide it. An examination of the patient's daily life will help us see how stressors can be reduced and the triggers that produce relapses avoided. The physician's continuing support will be an important factor in the process. Note how this approach transcends dualisms by ministering to the needs of the whole person. Our therapy is not divisible into biological or psychological or social. It is all three together. We have switched attention from the linear notions of cause and cure to the holistic notions of function, care, context, support, and healing.

The Need for a New Vocabulary

It will be difficult to change to a new way of thinking if we continue to use the old language of dualism. A new wine requires new wineskins. The old terminology forces us to think in dualistic terms. Is it really necessary to use terms like *psychosomatic, psychosocial,* and *biomedical* because they are based on the assumption that patients can be separated neatly into two components? This question leads naturally to the idea that we work along parallel lines, taking first a medical, then a social, history. It also leads to a distinction between "doing" therapies and "talking" therapies and between teaching biomedicine and psychosocial medicine. These ways of thinking are contrary to the responsiveness the patient-centered method enjoins. Using unifying terms such as *meaning, function,* and *care* encourages us to transcend these boundaries. If we ask whether an elderly widow with poor vision can take her medications, we are thinking in terms of a dosette box and a reminder phone call from her daughter; minimizing the number of drugs and the frequency of dose; and either improving her vision or putting instructions in large type. Caring for patients is attending to particulars, not dividing people into compartments. None of this need imply that we cease to categorize some therapy as behavioral, some as physical. But there is no need for this to be along binary lines. Let us be specific, calling it precisely what it is: cognitive, radiotherapeutic, pharmaceutical, psychoanalytical, supportive, relaxation, exercise, and so on.

It is interesting to note that some of the allied health disciplines have an orientation similar to this. Nursing bases its body of knowledge on the needs of persons, and physiotherapy and occupational therapy on function. Some recent movements in medicine also have transcended the divide: Approaches to rehabilitation and the management of chronic pain are in terms of function, rather than disease; and in palliative care, the focus is on the control of symptoms, whatever their origin. These trends, however, are outside the mainstream of medicine and medical education.

The Difficulties of Change

It is important not to underestimate the magnitude of the changes implied by the transformation of our clinical method. It is not simply a matter of learning some new techniques, though that is part of it. Nor is it only a question of adding courses in interviewing and behavioral science to the curriculum. The change goes much deeper than that. It requires nothing less than a change in what it means to be a physician, a different way of thinking about health and disease, and a redefinition of medical knowledge.

A glance at any medical school curriculum is usually sufficient to show that it is dominated by the modern paradigm of knowledge. Of course, this kind of knowledge is important, but restoring the balance in medicine requires that it be balanced by other kinds of knowledge: an understanding of human experience and human relationships, moral insight, and—that most difficult of accomplishments—self-knowledge. Much of this is not the kind of knowledge that can be learned in the classroom or from books, though some of it can. There is now, for example, a rich literature describing personal experiences of illness. If we are to give as much attention to care as we give to diagnosis, we will need to feed our imagination with accounts of what it is like to go blind, have multiple sclerosis, suffer bereavement, bring up a child with a disability, and the many other experiences our patients live with. We also will need to know the many practical ways in which life for them can be enriched or made more tolerable.

Human relationships and moral insight are not principally class-room subjects, except insofar as students learn moral lessons from the way they are treated by their teachers. However, once its importance is acknowledged and time is allowed for it, understanding of relationships can be deepened with the help of teachers who are sensitive, reflective, and prepared to expose their own vulnerability. Self-knowledge, by definition, cannot be taught. But its growth can be fostered by teachers who themselves are embarked on this difficult journey—a journey that is never complete.

Whitehead (1975) criticized professional education for being too full of abstractions, a condition he described as "the celibacy of the intellect" (p. 223), the modern equivalent of the celibacy of the medieval learned class. Wisdom, he believed, is the fruit of a balanced development. What we need is not more abstractions, but an education in which the necessary abstractions are balanced by concrete experiences, an education that feeds both the intellect and the imagination.

All of this implies that we see ourselves no longer as detached observers and dispassionate dispensers of therapy. To be patient-centered means to be open to a patient's feelings. It means becoming involved in a way that was made difficult by the old method. This has the potential for making medicine a much richer experience for us, as well as more effective for our patients. But beware the pitfalls. There are right and wrong ways of becoming involved. There are ways of dealing with some of the disturbing things our new openness will expose us to. Hence, the importance of the knowledge and insight I have already referred to.

The change we have to make is illustrated by the following example of a patient's experience with failing vision due to macular degeneration. The fact that the example is taken from ophthalmology does not imply that ophthalmologists were at fault; they were only practicing according to the conventional paradigm of medicine—as we all do.

The patient—a physician himself—described his experience.

> Through all of these years and despite many encounters with skilled and experienced professionals, no ophthalmologist has at any time suggested any devices that might be of assistance to me. No ophthalmologist has mentioned any of the many ways in which I could stem the deterioration in the quality of my life. Fortunately, I have discovered a number of means whereby I have helped myself, and the purpose of this essay is to call the attention of the ophthalmological world to some of these devices and, courteously but firmly, to complain of what appears to be the ophthalmologist's attitude: We are interested in vision but have little interest in blindness. (Stetten, 1981, p. 458)

Here, we see a failure of comprehension between two worlds. The patient, faced with the prospect of blindness, has to reconstruct his world, change it from one he constructed by using his five senses to one constructed through his remaining senses of touch, hearing, smell, and taste. Using the word *construct* recognizes that our "worlds" are not made from raw sensory data, but rather from how we interpret these data in the act of perception. Although our individual worlds have much in common, there are differences among individuals, among cultures and subcultures. The world of the blind is different from the world of the sighted.

It appears that the world constructed by the ophthalmologists included retinas and visual tests, but not the experience of becoming blind. To help the patient reconstruct his world, a physician would need to have some feeling for the suffering involved and enough imagination to empathize with the experience. Because the process of reconstruction will be different for each individual, the physician will need to attend to the particulars of each case. For example, one patient similarly afflicted had a lifelong interest in medieval cathedrals. Losing his vision made him experience cathedrals in a different way, through the effects of structure on sound and the exploration of shape by touch, rather than sight. His own experience led him to produce cathedral guides for the blind by using audiotapes and scale models that could be explored with the hands (Hull, 1992).

This example shows that if we are to recapture our capacity to heal, we will have to transcend the literal-mindedness that seems to follow when we become prisoners of our abstractions. A new clinical method should find room for the exercise of imagination and for restoring the balance between thinking and feeling.

A Different Way of Thinking About Health and Disease

Most difficult of all, perhaps, will be the transition from linear, causal thinking to cybernetic thinking. Linear thinking is deeply ingrained in our culture. The notion of a cause is based on the Newtonian model of a force acting on a passive object, as when a moving billiard ball hits a stationary one. The action is in one direction only. In medicine, this notion is exemplified by the doctrine of *specific etiology*—of an environmental agent acting on a person to produce a diseased state.

The notion of *cybernetic causation* is based on the model of self-organizing systems. The human organism can be viewed as a self-organizing system, maintaining itself by interaction with its environment and by a system of feedback loops from the environment and from its own output. Self-organizing systems have the ability to renew and transcend themselves. Healing is an example of self-renewal in which components are renewed while the integrity of the organization is maintained. Organisms transcend themselves by learning, developing, and growing. Self-organizing systems require energy, but as organizations they are maintained and changed by information. The notion of cause in self-organizing systems is based on the model of information that triggers a process that is already a potential of the system. The response is not the direct result of the original stimulus, but the result of rule-governed behavior that is a property of the system. If the process is long term, destabilizing, and self-perpetuating, then the question of cause becomes much more complex than that of identifying the trigger. The trigger that initiated the process may be quite different from the processes that perpetuate it. We must consider the processes in the organism that are perpetuating the disturbance. The key to enhancing healing may be in strengthening the organism's defenses, changing the information flow, or encouraging self-transcendence, rather than neutralizing an agent.

The Justification

Our modern dedication to instrumental knowledge requires that any change in what we do be justified by its effects. Does the patient-centered method improve patients' health? There is good evidence that it does. But I believe we are mistaken if we make this its justification. Some things are good in themselves. The justification of the patient-centered method is its moral basis.

Medicine has perennial moral problems, two of which are particularly serious in the present age: insensitivity to suffering and abuse of power. The distancing produced by our abstractions makes us especially prone to the first; our greatly enhanced prognostic and therapeutic power makes us especially liable to the second. Reforming our clinical method has at its deepest level a moral purpose: a restoration of the balance between thinking and feeling and a renunciation, or at least a sharing, of the enormous power modern technology has given us.

PART ONE

The Concepts

2

Overview of the Patient-Centered Clinical Method

W. WAYNE WESTON

JUDITH BELLE BROWN

Models of Medical Practice

Many colleges and academic associations of medicine have defined the knowledge, skills, and attitudes of the effective doctor. But these fall short of describing, in practical terms, the uniqueness of the doctor's clinical method. As medical professionals, we need a way to explain, clearly and pragmatically, the clinical tasks of medicine (White, 1988). Models of practice are valuable in several ways. First, they guide our perceptions by drawing our attention to specific features of practice. Second, they provide a framework for understanding what is going on. Third, they guide our actions by defining what is important. A productive model will not only simplify the complexity of reality but also focus our attention on aspects of a situation that are most important for understanding and effective action. The dominant model in medical practice today has been labeled the "conventional medical model." No one would question the widespread influence of the conventional medical model, but it often has been attacked for oversimplifying the problems of sickness (Odegaard, 1986; White, 1988). Engel (1977) described the problems with the conventional medical model this way:

It assumes disease to be fully accounted for by deviations from the norm of measurable biological (somatic) variables. It leaves no room within its framework for the social, psychological, and behavioral dimensions of illness. The biomedical model not only requires that disease be dealt with as an entity independent of social behaviour, it also demands that behavioral aberrations be explained on the basis of disordered somatic (biochemical or neurophysiological) processes. (p. 130)

In the past few years, a number of alternative conceptual frameworks have been recommended (Carmichael & Carmichael, 1981; Cohen-Cole, 1991; Foss & Rothenberg, 1987; Kleinman, Eisenberg, & Good, 1978; Pendleton et al., 1984). Engel's biopsychosocial model has attracted much attention. Engel (1980) uses systems theory as a basis for understanding human sickness. The patient is conceptualized as being composed of systems (tissues, cells, molecules) and, in turn, as being part of several larger systems (dyads, families, communities, nations). This model is valuable in reminding us to consider the personal and social dimensions of illness, in addition to biological aberrations. Yet, the model does not explain when or how to include these other dimensions. All of these conceptual models have been informative, have moved the practice of medicine forward, and have served as antecedents to our current work. However, an effective model of practice will need to be explicit about when and how to go beyond the conventional medical model.

Several authors (Hurowitz, 1993; Illich, 1976) have challenged an expanded model of medicine as unrealistic and arrogant: It is inappropriate to medicalize all human suffering and to expect physicians to find solutions to problems that have their origins in poverty, greed, racism, or ignorance. At the end of a 100-hour week, this argument has a certain appeal! But the debate ignores the reality of practice— that patients present to their doctors when they feel ill, no matter what the cause. At least, the physician must identify the source of the patient's distress and recommend appropriate resources for additional help. Furthermore, even treatment of organic disease may be ineffective if the patient's context is dismissed (e.g., family strife, unemployment, cultural differences). /

Other authors have pointed out the importance of acknowledging a distinction between the physician's theoretical understanding of the patient's disease and the patient's firsthand experience of feeling unwell (Cassell, 1985b, 1991; Fabrega, 1974; Levenstein, 1984; Levenstein et al., 1986; Levenstein et al., 1989; McWhinney, 1989b; Mishler, 1984; Reiser & Schroder, 1980; Stephens, 1982; Stetten, 1981). This distinction highlights patients' need for more than a scientific formulation and treatment of their problems. Patients generally want to feel understood and valued and to be involved in making sense of their health problems. In addition, many of them want to be involved in decisions about management.

A model of medicine will need to integrate the conventional understanding of disease with each patient's unique experience of illness. The patient-centered model presented in this book is an attempt to meet this need (Levenstein, 1984).

The patient-centered model is valuable in several ways:

1. It defines what doctors do when they are functioning well in helping their patients. It is not simply a model for curriculum or course planning, but rather a conceptual framework to guide the practitioner "in the trenches." Because the model is explicit about the behavior of an effective doctor, it provides a vocabulary and a focus for teaching and learning. The model provides more than a moral exhortation to be more caring; it provides a description of the specific behaviors that need to be learned, as well as guidelines about when and how to use them with patients. We call this description of specific behaviors "the method" that operationalizes the model.

2. The model is a reasonable representation of reality; it simplifies the complexity of the doctor's job without distorting it. Because the model grew out of medical practice, in particular, Dr. Levenstein's practice (Levenstein, 1984), rather than being imported from other disciplines, it has immediate applicability for experienced physicians.

3. The model applies to the majority of "ordinary" interactions between doctors and their patients.

4. The model provides a framework for research. By defining effective doctoring in discrete and measurable terms, specific components of practice can be evaluated.

The Patient-Centered Clinical Method

The term "patient-centered medicine" was introduced by Balint and colleagues (Balint, Hunt, Joyce, Marinker, & Woodcock, 1970),

who contrasted it with "illness-centered medicine." An understanding of the patient's complaints, based on patient-centered thinking, was called "overall diagnosis," and an understanding based on
disease-centered thinking was called "traditional diagnosis." The
clinical method was elaborated by Stevens (1974) and Tait (1979).
Byrne and Long (1976) developed a method for categorizing a consultation as doctor-centered or patient-centered, their concept of a
doctor-centered consultation being close to other writers' "illness"- or
"disease"-centered methods. Wright and MacAdam (1979) also described doctor-centered and patient-centered clinical methods. A
patient-centered clinical method has much in common with the psychotherapeutic concept of client-centered therapy (Rogers, 1951), with
Newman and Young's (1972) total-person approach to patient problems in nursing, and with the two-body practice in occupational
therapy (Mattingly & Fleming, 1994).

Byrne and Long (1976), in their analysis of 1,850 general practice
consultations, suggested that many physicians develop a relatively
static style of consulting that tends to be doctor-centered: "The problem is that the doctor-centered style is extremely seductive" (p. 125).
Clinical teaching in medical schools tends to emphasize a doctor-
centered approach (or disease-centered, as we prefer). According to
this model, physicians ascertain the patient's complaints and seek
information that will enable them to interpret the patient's illness
within their own frame of reference. This involves diagnosing the
patient's disease and prescribing an appropriate management. One
criterion of success is a precise diagnosis, such as myocardial infarction, stroke, carcinoma of the colon, child abuse, attempted suicide, or alcoholism. In pursuit of this goal, physicians use a method
designed to obtain objective information from the patient.

In this chapter, we briefly describe the patient-centered model and
method developed by Levenstein (1984) in his own practice and
further developed at The University of Western Ontario (Levenstein,
McCracken, McWhinney, Stewart, & Brown, 1986; McCracken, Stewart,
Brown, & McWhinney, 1983). The model consists of six interconnect-
ing components, summarized in Table 2.1 and illustrated in Figure
2.1, each of which is described in more detail in Chapters 3 through 8:

1. Exploring both the disease and the illness experience
2. Understanding the whole person

TABLE 2.1 The Patient-Centered Clinical Method

The six interactive components of the patient-centered process:

1. Exploring both the disease and the illness experience
   A. Differential diagnosis
   B. Dimensions of illness (ideas, feelings, expectations, and effects on function)
2. Understanding the whole person
   A. The "person" (life history and personal and developmental issues)
   B. The context (the family and anyone else involved in or affected by the patient's illness; the physical environment)
3. Finding common ground regarding management
   A. Problems and priorities
   B. Goals of treatment
   C. Roles of doctor and patient in management
4. Incorporating prevention and health promotion
   A. Health enhancement
   B. Risk reduction
   C. Early detection of disease
   D. Ameliorating effects of disease
5. Enhancing the patient-doctor relationship
   A. Characteristics of the therapeutic relationship
   B. Sharing power
   C. Caring and healing relationship
   D. Self-awareness
   E. Transference and countertransference
6. Being realistic
   A. Time
   B. Resources
   C. Team building

3. Finding common ground
4. Incorporating prevention and health promotion
5. Enhancing the patient-doctor relationship
6. Being realistic

1. EXPLORING BOTH THE DISEASE AND THE ILLNESS EXPERIENCE

The first component involves physicians' understanding two conceptualizations of ill health with all of their patients: disease and illness (Levenstein, 1984; Levenstein et al., 1986; Levenstein et al.,

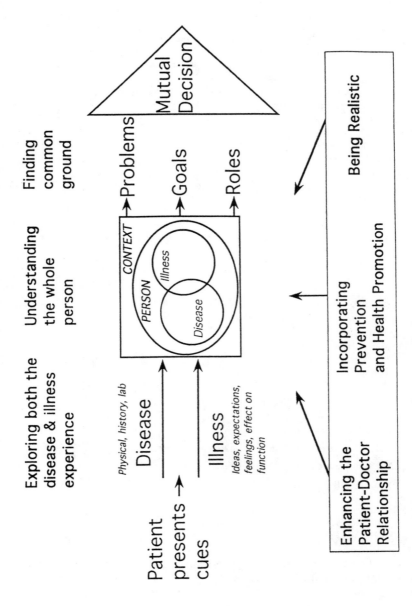

Figure 2.1. The Patient-Centered Clinical Method.

1989). *Disease* is a theoretical construct, or abstraction, by which physicians attempt to explain patients' problems in terms of abnormalities of structure and/or function of body organs and systems and includes both physical and mental disorders. *Illness* refers to patients' personal experiences of ill health. The diagnostic label explains what each individual with a disease has in common with all others, but the illness of each person is unique.

Effective patient care requires attending as much to patients' personal experiences of illnesses as to their diseases. The identification of disease is established by using the conventional medical model, but understanding illnesses requires an additional approach. A patient-centered method focuses on disease and on four principal dimensions of patients' illness experiences: (a) their ideas about what is wrong with them; (b) their feelings, especially fears about being ill; (c) the impact of their problems on functioning; and (d) their expectations about what should be done. The key to this approach is attention to patients' cues related to these dimensions; the goal is to follow patients' leads, to understand patients' experiences from their own points of view. This method improves patient satisfaction, compliance, and outcomes of both illness and disease and is applicable to the everyday work of physicians with "ordinary" patients.

Reaching a therapeutic understanding of patients' illness experiences requires skill in interviewing to enable the doctor to "enter into the patient's world," to understand the illness from the patient's point of view. Often this component will be straightforward; at other times, however, the doctor must be alert for any cues to the patient's ideas, expectations, feelings, or effects on function. Patients may prompt a doctor if he or she misses cues. Sometimes, it is only at the end of an interview that a crucial comment is made. These "doorknob" remarks may indicate that the doctor has missed earlier cues or that the patient finally has summoned up enough courage to raise a fearful or embarrassing issue before it is too late.

2. UNDERSTANDING THE WHOLE PERSON

The second component is an integrated understanding of the whole person. Over time, doctors accumulate a myriad of information about their patients that goes beyond diagnosing disease or attending to illness responses. They begin to know the whole person and, in doing so, come to understand the patient's disease and experience of illness in the context of his or her life setting and stage of personal development. This knowledge of the person may include the family, work, beliefs, and struggles with various life crises.

Serious illness of a family member reverberates throughout the entire family system. The doctor who understands the whole person recognizes the impact of the family in ameliorating, aggravating, or even causing illness in its members. The patient's cultural beliefs and attitudes also influence his or her care.

An understanding of the whole person can enhance the physician's interaction with the patient at specific times—for example, when the signs or symptoms do not point to a clearly defined disease process or when the patient's response to an illness appears exaggerated or out of character. On these occasions, consideration of the patient's position in the life cycle may shed some light on his or her current experience. But even when the diagnosis is clear and uncomplicated, knowledge of the whole person can help the doctor answer the question "Why now?"

Finally, understanding the whole person can deepen the doctor's knowledge of the human condition, especially the nature of suffering and the responses of persons to sickness.

3. FINDING COMMON GROUND

The third component of the method is the mutual undertaking of finding common ground. Developing an effective management plan requires physician and patient to reach agreement in three key areas: (a) the nature of the problems and priorities, (b) the goals of treatment, and (c) the roles of the doctor and the patient. Often, doctors and patients have widely divergent views in each of these areas. The process of finding a satisfactory resolution is not so much one of bargaining or negotiating, but rather of moving toward a meeting of minds or finding common ground. This framework reminds physicians to incorporate patients' ideas, feelings, expectations, and function into treatment planning.

4. INCORPORATING PREVENTION AND HEALTH PROMOTION

The fourth component incorporates prevention and health promotion into the context of the "ordinary" office visit. As disease prevention and health promotion require a collaborative, ongoing effort on the part of patient and physician, the process of finding common ground on the multiplicity of opportunities for disease prevention and health promotion becomes an important component of every visit. Application of the patient-centered approach throughout this process constitutes health promotion as currently defined (World Health Organization, 1986a)—that is, "the process of enabling people to take control over and to improve their health" (p. 73).

Within such a supportive process, physicians and patients together monitor areas in patients' lives that need strengthening in the interests of long-term emotional and physical health. Physicians also need to monitor recognized problems and to screen for unrecognized disease. Finally, physicians need to collaborate with other health professionals to implement the program of health promotion and screening in practice.

This task requires that continuing and comprehensive care is the underlying philosophy of·the practice and that a protocol for screening and health promotion, as well as a medical record system that supports the protocol (e.g., problem list, flow sheets, tickler files, computer reminder systems), be implemented.

5. ENHANCING THE PATIENT-DOCTOR RELATIONSHIP

The fifth component of the patient-centered method is conscious attention to enhancing the patient-doctor relationship. When doctors see the same patients time after time with a variety of problems, they acquire considerable personal knowledge of them that may be helpful in managing subsequent problems. At every visit, in the context of continuity of care, physicians strive to build an effective long-term relationship with each patient as a foundation for their work together and to use the relationship for its healing potential. Physicians (using personal self-awareness, as well as the basic tools of effective relationships: unconditional positive regard, empathy, and genuineness) attend fully to patients and their needs without always having to interpret or intervene. Physicians recognize that different patients require different approaches and use themselves in a variety of ways to meet the patients' needs (e.g., sensing a patient who has unquenchable need for support and is vulnerable to abandonment; recognizing and accommodating an assertive, involved patient). Physicians, at the very least, "walk with" the patients and, at most, use themselves and their relationship to mobilize the strengths of patients for a healing purpose.

6. BEING REALISTIC

The sixth component involves being realistic. Doctors frequently have competing demands for their time and energy; they must learn to manage their time efficiently for the maximum benefit of their patients. Physicians must develop skills of priority setting, resource allocation, and teamwork. Doctors practicing in primary care settings are the providers of first entry into the health care system and, as such, must be wise stewards of the community's resources. Finally, doctors must respect their own limits of emotional energy and not expect too much of themselves.

Conclusion

Although the six interactive components of the patient-centered clinical method have been presented as separate and discrete, in reality the components are intricately interwoven. The skilled clinician moves effortlessly back and forth, following the patients' cues, among the six components. We have found this technique of weaving back and forth to be a key concept in teaching the method and one that requires practice and experience.

3

The First Component

Exploring Both the
Disease and the Illness Experience

JUDITH BELLE BROWN

W. WAYNE WESTON

MOIRA STEWART

The first component of the patient-centered clinical method was demonstrated and described to the authors by Dr. Joseph Levenstein (1984, 1986, 1989). The basis of this method is a distinction between two conceptualizations of ill health: disease and illness. Effective patient care requires attending as much to patients' personal experiences of illnesses as to their diseases. Diseases are diagnosed by using the conventional medical model, but understanding illnesses requires a different approach. *Disease,* on the one hand, is an abstraction, the "thing" that is wrong with the body-as-machine. *Illness,* on the other hand, is the patient's personal experience of sickness—the thoughts, feelings, and altered behavior of someone who feels sick.

In the biomedical model, sickness is explained in terms of pathophysiology: abnormal structure and function of tissues and organs.

AUTHORS' NOTE: Parts of this chapter were published previously in *Canadian Family Physician* (1989), 35, 147-151.

This model is a conceptual framework for understanding the biological dimensions of sickness by reducing sickness to disease. The focus is on the body, not on the person. A particular disease is what everyone with that disease has in common, but the illness experience of each person is unique. Disease and illness do not always coexist. Patients with undiagnosed asymptomatic disease are not ill; people who are grieving or worried may feel ill but have no disease. Patients and doctors who recognize this distinction and who realize how common it is to feel ill and have no disease are less likely to search needlessly and fruitlessly for pathology. Even when disease is present, however, it may not adequately explain the patient's suffering, because the amount of distress a patient experiences refers not only to the amount of tissue damage but to the personal meaning of the illness.

Several authors have described this same distinction between disease and illness from different perspectives. In analyzing medical interviews, Mishler (1984) identified two contrasting voices: the voice of medicine and the voice of the lifeworld. The voice of medicine, on the one hand, promotes a scientific, detached attitude and uses such questions as, "Where does it hurt?" "When did it start?" "How long does it last?" "What makes it better or worse?" The voice of the lifeworld, on the other hand, reflects a "common sense" view of the world. It centers on the individual's particular social context, the meaning of illness events, and how these may affect the achievement of personal goals. Typical questions to ask in exploring the lifeworld are "What are you most concerned about?" "How does it disrupt your life?" "What do you think it is?" "How do you think I can help you?"

Mishler (1984) argued that typical interactions between doctors and patients are doctor centered; they are dominated by a technocratic perspective. The physician's task is to make a diagnosis; thus, in the interview, the doctor selectively attends to the voice of medicine, often not even hearing patients' own attempts to make sense of their suffering. What is needed is a different approach in which doctors give priority to "patients' lifeworld contexts of meaning as the basis for understanding, diagnosing and treating their problems" (Mishler, 1984, p. 192).

Eric Cassell (1985b) has a corresponding message:

> The story of an illness—the patient's history—has two protagonists: the body and the person. By careful questioning, it is possible to separate

out the facts that speak of disturbed bodily functioning, the pathophysi-ology that gives you the diagnosis. To do this, the facts about the body's dysfunction must be separated from the meanings that the patient has attached to them. Skillful physicians have been doing this for ages. All too often, however, the personal meanings are then discarded. With them goes the doctor's opportunity to know who the patient is. (p. 108)

Kleinman and others have described an ethnomedical model based on their work in anthropology (Galazka & Eckert, 1986; Katon & Kleinman, 1981; Kleinman et al., 1978). This model emphasizes the importance of eliciting patients' "explanatory models" of their ill-nesses and offers a series of questions to ask patients that they call a "cultural status exam." The physician might ask, for example: "How would you describe the problem that has brought you to me?" "Does anyone else you know have these problems?" "What do you think is causing the problem?" "Why do you think this problem has happened to you, and why now?" "What do you think will clear up this prob-lem?" "Apart from me, who else do you think can help you get better?" (Good & Good, 1981).

Several studies in primary care demonstrate the inadequacy of the conventional medical model for explaining many of the problems patients bring to their doctors. Blacklock (1977) found that in 50% of 109 patients who presented to their family physicians with chest pain, the etiology was unproven after 6-month follow-up. In Jerritt's (1981) study of 300 patients who complained of lethargy, fatigue, or tired-ness, no organic cause could be found in 62.3% of patients, who were evaluated in a general practice during a 3-year period. Wasson, Sox, and Sox (1981), investigating 525 unselected male patients with ab-dominal pain who presented to an outpatient clinic, found no evi-dence for specific organic diagnosis in 79%.

Several authors (Morrell, 1972; Peabody, 1927; Research Committee of the College of General Practitioners, 1958) have suggested that in only half of all patients presenting to a family doctor can the physician find a disease to explain the patient's problem. Rarely is this lack because the disease is hidden; most often, it is because the patient's feelings of ill health have their source in other factors: an unhappy marriage, job dissatisfaction, guilt, or lack of purpose in life. In a study of housewives who kept health diaries, Freer (1980) found that this group of women frequently described "symptoms" such as headaches, feeling tired and run down, or various aches and pains. Most of these complaints they handled on their own by resting or putting up with them. Many women reported that doing housework or going shopping made them feel better. For only 1 out of 40 complaints did they seek medical advice.

The number of times in a year a person visits a doctor varies tremendously, depending on the doctor, the social class, and the country. It would be difficult to explain these differences on the basis of disease prevalence; social and cultural factors have a stronger influence on help-seeking behavior than has symptom severity. This may be one reason why hospital-trained physicians become frustrated with primary care. However, it does not take long for primary care physicians to realize that a strictly biomedical approach to illness is ineffective. This realization highlights the importance of having additional approaches to understanding human sickness.

The Stages of Illness

The reasons patients present themselves to a doctor when they do are often more important than the diagnosis. Frequently, the diagnosis is obvious or already is known from previous contacts; often, no biomedical label can explain a patient's problem. Thus it is often more helpful to answer the question "Why now?" than the question "What's the diagnosis?" In chronic illness, for example, a change in a social situation is a more common reason for presenting than a change in the disease or the symptoms.

The illness experience has several stages. Illness is often a painful crisis that will overwhelm the coping abilities of some patients and challenge others to increased personal growth. It is helpful to understand these reactions as part of a developmental process that has three stages: awareness, disorganization, and reorganization (Reiser & Schroder, 1980). The first stage, *awareness*, is characterized by ambivalence about knowing: on the one hand, wanting to know the truth and to understand the illness, and on the other, not wanting to admit that anything could be wrong. At the same time, patients often are struggling with conflicting wishes to remain independent and longings to be taken care of. Eventually, if the symptoms do not go away, the fact of the illness hits home and patients' sense of being in control of their own lives is shattered.

This shattering disrupts the universal defense: the magical belief that somehow we are immune from disease, injury, and death. The patient who has struggled to forestall his or her awareness of serious illness and then finally has recognized the truth is one of the most fragile, defenseless, and exquisitely vulnerable people one can ever find. This is a time of terror and depression (Reiser & Schroder, 1980).

At this second stage, *disorganization*, patients typically regress to childhood defenses and react to their caretakers as parents, rather than as equals. They often become self-centered and demanding, and although they may be aware of this reaction and embarrassed by it, they cannot seem to stop it. They may withdraw from the external world and become preoccupied with each little change in their bodies. Their sense of time becomes constricted, and the future seems uncertain; they may lose a sense of continuity of self. They can no longer trust their bodies, and they feel diminished and out of control. Their whole sense of their personal identities may be severely threatened. One reaction to this state of mind in some patients is rebellion, a desperate attempt to have at least some small measure of control over their lives even if it is self-destructive in the end.

In the third stage, *reorganization*, patients call on all of their inner strength to find new meaning in the face of illness and, if possible, to transcend their plight. Their degree of mastery will be affected, of course, by the nature and severity of the illness. But in addition, the outcome is profoundly influenced by the patients' social supports, especially loving relationships within their families, and by the type of support their physician can provide.

These stages of illness are part of a normal human response to disaster, and not another set of disease categories or psychopathology. This description emphasizes how the humanity of the ill person is compromised and points to an added obligation of physicians to their wounded patients.

So great is the assault of illness upon our being that "it is almost as if our natures themselves were ill, as if the strands or parts of us were being forced apart and we verged on the loss of our own humanness." A phenomenon so great in its effects that it can threaten us with the loss of our fundamental humanness clearly requires more than technical competence from those who would "treat" illness. (Kestenbaum, 1982, pp. viii-ix)

Four Dimensions
of the Illness Experience

Patients often provide physicians with cues and prompts about the reason they are coming to the physician that day. These may be verbal or nonverbal signals. The patients may look tearful, sigh deeply, or be short of breath. They may say directly, "I feel awful, Doctor. I think this flu is going to kill me." Or, indirectly, they may present a variety of vague symptoms that are masking a more serious illness, such as depression. As doctors sit down with patients and ask, "What brings you in today?" they must ask themselves, "What has precipitated this visit?"

We propose four dimensions of illness experience that physicians should explore: (a) patients' ideas about what is wrong; (b) their feelings, especially their fears, about their problems; (c) their expectations of the doctor; and (d) the effect of the illness on functioning (Weston, Brown, & Stewart, 1989; see Figure 3.1). When physicians address these aspects of illness, patients are more likely to be satisfied with their doctors, more likely to comply with the treatment recommendations, and more likely to recover (Stewart et al., 1989).

What are the patients' *ideas* about their illness? What meaning do they attach to the illness experience? Many persons endure illness as an irreparable loss; others may view it as an opportunity to gain valuable insight into their life experience. Is the illness seen as a form of punishment or, perhaps, as an opportunity for dependency? Whatever the illness, knowing its meaning is paramount for understanding the patient.

What are the patients' *feelings?* Do the patients fear that the symptoms they present may be the precursor of a more serious problem, such as cancer? Some patients may feel a sense of relief and view the illness as an opportunity for respite from demands or responsibilities. Patients often feel angry or guilty about being ill.

What are their *expectations* of the doctor? Does the presentation of a sore throat carry with it an expectation of penicillin? Do they want the doctor to do something or just listen?

What are the effects of the illness on *function?* Does it limit patients' daily activities? Does it impair their family relationships? Does it require a change in lifestyle?

The following examples of patient-doctor dialogue contain specific questions that physicians might ask to elicit this information.

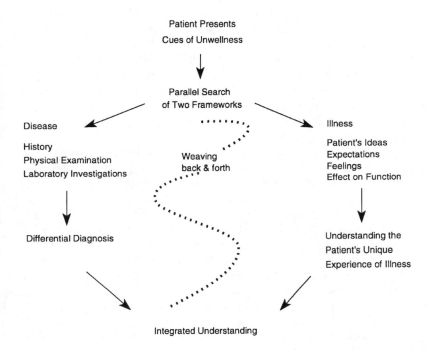

Figure 3.1. The Patient-Centered Clinical Method.

To the doctor's question, "What brings you in today?" a patient responds, "I've had these severe headaches for the last few weeks. I'm wondering if there is something I can do about them." To examine the patient's ideas about the headaches, the physician might ask (waiting after each question for the patient's reply): "What do you think is causing the headaches?" "Have you any ideas or theories about why you might be having them?" "Do you think there is any relationship between the headaches and current events in your life?"

The patient's feelings about the headaches can be elicited by such questions as, "What are your concerns about the headache?" "Do you think something sinister is causing them?" "Is something particularly worrisome for you about the headaches?"

To determine how the headaches may be impeding the patient's function, the doctor might ask, "How are your headaches affecting your day-to-day living?" "Are they stopping you from participating in any activities?" "Is there any connection between the headaches and the way your life is going?"

Finally, to identify the patient's expectations of the physician at this visit, the doctor might inquire, "What do you think would help you deal with these headaches?" "Is there some specific management that you want for your headaches?" "In what way may I help you?" "Have you a particular test in mind?" "What do you think would reassure you about these headaches?"

Certain illnesses or events in the lives of individuals may cause them embarrassment or emotional discomfort. As a result, patients may not always feel at ease with themselves or their physician and may cloak their primary concerns in a myriad of symptoms. The doctor must, on occasion, respond to each of these symptoms to create an environment in which patients may feel more trusting and comfortable about exposing their concerns. Often, the doctor will provide them with an avenue to express their feelings by commenting, "I sense that something is troubling you or that something more is going on. Can I help you with that?"

Identifying the key questions to be asked should not be taken lightly. Malterud (1994) described a method for clinicians to formulate and evaluate the wording of key questions. The wording of questions should be comfortable for the doctor and suited to the patient's context.

The following case example provides an illustration of the patient-centered method:

CASE EXAMPLE

Mr. R., 58 years of age, had been a patient in the practice for 10 years. Until 8 months ago, when he had a massive myocardial infarction and required triple coronary artery bypass surgery, he had been a healthy man with few problems. He was married, with grown children, and had returned to work as a plumber. He had come to the office for diet counseling about his elevated cholesterol.

The following excerpt from the visit demonstrates the doctor's use of the patient-centered approach. The interaction began with the doctor stating, "So, Mr. R., you're in about your diet. Looks like your cholesterol levels are dropping nicely." "Yes," responded Mr. R. "That's good news, and I'm feeling pretty good about my weight. I'm down 5 more pounds and almost at my goal." The doctor proceeded to explore Mr. R.'s diet in some detail.

The interview then shifted to Mr. R.'s weight-loss program, and he stated that he had been dutifully following his exercise regimen throughout the summer months and was walking up to 4 miles a day. The doctor asked, "Will you be able to continue your walking during the winter?"

"Oh yes," indicated Mr. R. "I don't mind walking in the winter. I quite enjoy it. I just have to be careful on those very cold days."

"Yes, you do need to be cautious during the severe weather," replied the doctor. Mr. R. looked away and appeared sad. The doctor paused and asked, "Is there something concerning you, Mr. R.?"

"Oh well . . . no," stated Mr. R. quickly. "No, not really."

"Not really?" reflected the doctor.

"Well," replied Mr. R., "I was just thinking about the winter and . . . well . . . no, I guess I'll be able to snowmobile if I just keep warm."

"Why are you concerned that you won't be able to do that, Mr. R.?" asked the doctor.

"Well, I don't know. I'd just miss it if I couldn't participate."

"It sounds as if that activity is important to you," responded the doctor.

"Well, yes, it has been a very important family activity. We have some land and a little cabin up north of here, and it's really how we spend our winter weekends—the whole family together."

"It sounds as if not being able to participate in something that's been an important family activity would be very difficult for you," reflected the doctor.

"Oh, yes, it would be. I just feel that so many things have been taken away from me that I really would miss not being able to do that."

The doctor responded, "Mr. R., it seems that in the last several months you have experienced a lot of changes and a lot of losses. I sense it has been very difficult for you."

"Yes, Doc, it has. It's been tough. I've gone from being a man who is really healthy and has no problems to having a bad heart attack and a big operation and being a real weight watcher. It has been a big change, and it has had its tough moments, but I'm alive and I guess that is what matters," answered Mr. R.

"It seems that you still have a lot of feelings surrounding your heart attack and the surgery and the changes that have occurred," commented the doctor.

"Yes, I have," Mr. R. replied soberly. "I have."

"Would it be helpful at some time for us to talk about that more, to set aside some time just to look at that?" inquired the doctor.

Mr. R. replied, "Yes it would. It's hard to talk about, but it would be helpful."

"Just briefly, are you encountering any problems with sleep or appetite?" asked the doctor.

"No, none at all," stated Mr. R.

The doctor asked a few more questions, exploring possible symptoms of depression. Finding none, he again offered to talk further with Mr. R. at their next visit. Mr. R. answered affirmatively.

In this example, the patient's situation can be summarized by using the disease and illness framework that is part of the patient-centered model illustrated in Figure 3.2.

The doctor already knew the patient's disorders before the interview began. He picked up on the patient's sadness and hesitancy in exploring how he was experiencing his illness. At the same time, the doctor ruled out serious depression by asking a few diagnostic questions and offered the patient an opportunity to explore further his feelings about his illness. The interview effortlessly weaved back and forth between the disease issues and the illness experience.

By considering the patient's illness experience as a legitimate focus of inquiry and management, the physician avoided two potential errors. First, if the conventional biomedical model only had been used, by seeking a disease to explain the patient's distress the doctor might have labeled the patient "depressed" and given him unnecessary and potentially hazardous medication. Second, the doctor could have concluded that the patient was not depressed. Had the physician decided that the patient's distress was normal, he may have considered the patient's concerns as not warranting further discussion.

This case also illustrates that doctors are often very limited in what they can do about a patient's disease. Lowering this man's cholesterol

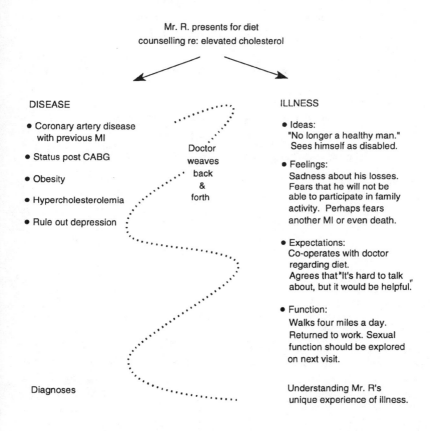

Figure 3.2. The Patient-Centered Method Applied.

is unlikely to have a great effect on his health after his disease has progressed so far. Dealing with this patient's experience of illness, however, may be helpful by alleviating fears, correcting misconceptions, encouraging him to discuss his discouragement, or simply by "being there" and caring what happens to him. At the very least, this compassionate concern is a testimony to the fundamental worth and dignity of the patient; it might help prevent him from becoming truly depressed; it might even help him live more fully.

BEING UNDERSTOOD

Case Illustrating Component 1:
Exploring Both the
Disease and the Illness Experience

Judith Belle Brown
W. Wayne Weston
Moira Stewart

My God, I can't see!

The patient was a 32-year-old male executive who suddenly went blind in his left eye while driving home from work with his wife and young daughter. The loss of vision had been preceded by severe pain around the eye for 48 hours, which the patient had attributed to stress at work. Now terrified by what was happening, he immediately sought medical attention. He was assessed initially by the ophthalmology team in the emergency department, subsequently referred to neurology, and then finally admitted to the hospital for investigation. For the next 10 anxious days, he underwent a thorough workup.

What made the intrusive examinations, the uncomfortable procedures, the pain of the illness, the uncertainty, and the blindness bearable to this young man was the medical team. Along with aggressively seeking the origin of his physical symptoms to establish a diagnosis, the doctors attended to the patient's personal experience of being sick. They heeded the four dimensions of the patient's illness experience: his ideas about his illness, his feelings, his expectations of what might be done, and the effect of the illness on his day-to-day functioning. For example, they discussed the patient's ideas about the illness: what it might be—a stroke, multiple sclerosis, or a brain tumor;

how it had originated; whether it was related to stress; and why the onset had been so sudden.

In addition, they dealt with his questions regarding the tests and their implications. They not only examined his physical pain but also attended to his emotional pain. His fear and anxiety were acknowledged and discussed. They did not dismiss his frustration or ignore his anger about "Why me?" By providing him with an opportunity to express his feelings, the doctors helped the patient make some sense of what was happening to him. The doctors not only observed the effect of the illness on his day-to-day functioning in the hospital but also discussed with him how this might affect his professional responsibilities and family life. Together, they explored options and alternatives, depending on the final diagnosis.

The patient's expectations of the physicians was that they would listen to him, answer his questions, provide him with the facts, and be available when needed. He found solace in their concern and appreciated their honesty and candor.

In brief, the medical team took the time to understand this man's illness by eliciting and allowing the expression of his ideas and feelings about the illness experience. They responded to his expectations and acknowledged the various implications of the illness on his roles as a professional, a husband, and a father.

The final diagnosis was optic neuritis, and there was a 90% return of the patient's vision. He continued to ask, "Why me?" and "How did this happen?" Yet, he felt comforted and supported by the medical team that responded to his ideas about his illness and cared about his fears and concerns. His expectations were that he would continue to be monitored by the team as required and that they would continue to be patient-centered.

NOTE: This case description first appeared in the May 1990 issue of the *Ontario Medical Review* and is reprinted with the permission of the Ontario Medical Association.

4

The Second Component

Understanding the Whole Person

JUDITH BELLE BROWN

W. WAYNE WESTON

In the previous chapter, we examined the importance of exploring both the disease and the illness experience, including their meaning for the patient. But disease and illness cannot be viewed in isolation. Patient-centered care includes understanding the person and the world in which he or she lives. Therefore the second component of the patient-centered clinical method is the integration of the concepts of disease and illness with an understanding of the whole person, including an awareness of the patient's position in the life cycle and his or her life context. The patient's position in the life cycle takes into consideration the individual's own personality development, as well as the family's various stages of development. The patient's life context includes his or her family, friendship networks, employment, school, religion, culture, and the health care system.

In this chapter, we discuss the interrelationship that exists among the disease, the illness, and the person who experiences them. This includes examining the person from the perspectives of both individual development and the family life cycle. In addition, we explore the

AUTHORS' NOTE: The authors thank Oxford University Press for permission to quote from E. J. Cassell (1991), *The nature of suffering and the goals of medicine*.

influence of the larger social system and culture in which patients live their lives.

The Person:
Individual Development

Multiple theoretical frameworks can help doctors understand patients' individual development and provide both explanation and prediction about patient behavior and responses to illness. For example, they include psychoanalytic theory (ego psychology, object relations, and self-psychology), feminist theory, and cognitive theory. A comprehensive overview of these various theoretical frameworks has been provided by numerous authors (e.g., Eagle, 1984; Erikson, 1950, 1982; Gilligan, 1982; Jordan, Kaplan, Miller, Stiver, & Surrey, 1991; Kohut, 1971, 1977; Mishne, 1993; Piaget, 1950). The intent of this section of the chapter is to highlight the importance of understanding individual development and to demonstrate how this can be achieved in the context of the patient-centered approach.

Understanding patients' diseases is only one dimension of their personhood. They are parents, partners, sons, and daughters who have a past, a present, and a future. The motives, attachments, ideals, and expectations that shape their personalities evolve as they negotiate each developmental phase. Healthy individual development is reflected by a solid sense of self, positive self-esteem, and a position of independence and autonomy, coupled with the capacity for connectedness and intimacy. Their lives are greatly influenced by each developmental phase, which may be isolated and lonely for an elderly widow or vast and complex for a middle-aged woman with multiple responsibilities as wife, mother, daughter, and worker. Thus their position in the life cycle, the tasks they assume, and the roles they ascribe to will influence the care that patients seek. As an illustration of the impact of illness on human development, consider the teenager, grappling with the demands of peer acceptance, who is ostracized because of his or her acne; or the middle-aged woman, coping with the empty-nest syndrome, who is reminded of her loss of fertility by the symptoms of menopause.

Understanding the patient's current stage of development and the relevant developmental tasks that need to be accomplished assist doctors in several ways. First, knowledge of the expectable life stage crises that occur in individual development help the doctor recognize the patient's problems as more than isolated, episodic phenomena. Second, it can increase the doctor's sensitivity to the multiple factors that influence the patient's problems and broaden awareness of the impact of the patient's life history. For example, the onset of a chronic illness at an early age may interfere with negotiation of age-specific tasks. Such is the case of juvenile onset diabetes, which may create difficulty for an adolescent attempting to negotiate the turbulent process of becoming independent. Third, understanding the whole person may expand the doctor's level of comfort with caring, as well as curing.

In the following case example, we observe how multiple losses throughout a patient's life had a powerful influence on the prospect of retirement, complicated by illness.

CASE EXAMPLE

The patient, age 55, had devoted herself to her career as a nurse. An early retirement option had provided her with the opportunity to pursue other interests, such as extended travel. But, without warning, she had been stricken with debilitating back pain that severely restricted her activities. She felt isolated, alone, and helpless. An only child, she had cared for her elderly parents throughout her 20s and 30s. Finally, "freed" by their deaths, she became involved in the first significant relationship in her life. After 5 years of marriage, her husband died of cancer when she was age 45. She then placed all of her energy and aspirations into her career. Her life revolved around her work and served as her major source of self-esteem. Her second love was travel, which never had been possible because of family and work commitments. Early retirement, she had hoped, would allow her to pursue this interest. Now faced with her loss of physical ability, coupled with her loss of status as a caregiver, the option of retirement seemed one of despair and loneliness. As her losses accumulated, she struggled to find meaning in her life, becoming progressively more depressed and physically incapacitated.

✧✧✧

An understanding of the whole person enhances the physician's interaction with the patient and may be particularly helpful when signs or symptoms do not point to a clearly defined disease process or when the patient's response to an illness appears exaggerated or out of character. On these occasions, it is often helpful to explore how the patient is dealing with the common issues related to his or her stage in the life cycle. Knowing that a patient has minimal family interaction or limited social support alerts the physician to an individual at risk. Also, being aware of prior losses or developmental crises assists the doctor in identifying vulnerable junctures in the patient's life.

The Person and the Family Life Cycle

A vast literature on family theory exists to explain and understand the intricacies and dynamics of family systems. It is not the purpose of this chapter to provide a comprehensive overview of this area, but rather to highlight the important role of the family in understanding the whole person. The reader is directed to texts that provide clear and thoughtful presentations of the family life cycle and family systems (Carter & McGoldrick, 1989; Hartman & Laird, 1983) and additional works that link family systems and primary care (Candib, 1985; Carmichael, 1973; Christie-Seely, 1984; Doherty & Baird, 1986; Fisher, Ransom, & Terry, 1993; McDaniel et al., 1990; Medalie, 1978; Ransom, 1993; Sawa, 1985; Smilkstein, 1978, 1984).

In concurrence with other authors (Carter & McGoldrick, 1989; Hartman & Laird, 1983; McDaniel et al., 1990), we define *family* as two or more people related or connected biologically, emotionally, or legally. Our conceptualization extends beyond the traditional notion of the family to encompass such unions as gay and lesbian couples, common-law relationships, single-parent families, couples without children, and households composed of friends. Although the composition and roles of the family have changed and expanded, the function of the family has remained constant: to provide a nurturing, safe, and continuous environment that promotes the physical, psychological, and social well-being of its members (Carmichael, 1978; Ransom & Vanderwoort, 1973; Woods & Hollis, 1990). In today's society, this is a daunting task. The family is buffeted by internal and external forces. The rising divorce rate, the increase in single-parent households, changes in traditional sex role relationships, and the reentry of women in the workforce challenge the function of the family. The health and well-being of families is assaulted by such problems as child and spousal abuse, suicide, AIDS, and substance abuse. Families also must face the enormous strain imposed by unemployment, poverty, and homelessness.

The additional burden of illness, either acute or chronic, may cause severe disruption to an already overtaxed family system (Mailick, 1979; Rolland, 1989). Illness is a powerful agent of change. The impact of illness on the family is as diverse as the devastating loss of the breadwinner role caused by a cardiovascular accident or the riveting effect on a family when a child is diagnosed with cerebral palsy. In other instances, the illness initially may appear superficial and benign, as demonstrated in the case of the young woman with a broken ankle (see "Lost Dreams: Case Illustrating Component 2" later in this chapter). Yet, the implications of her sports injury had a significant impact on her sense of self and her family relationships.

Illness in the family causes a major disruption that alters how family members relate and ultimately may impede their ability to overcome the ramifications of the illness experience. Illness may demand a change in the family role structure and task allocation. Changes in routine, such as child care responsibilities or visits to the hospital, may be required. Major alterations, such as substantial home renovations to accommodate a wheelchair-bound family member or a return to the workforce to provide for the financial needs of the family, may be needed.

The family disequilibrium resulting from illness also can alter the established rules and expectations of the family members, transform their methods of communication, and substantially alter the family structure. For example, after the diagnosis of terminal breast cancer, a mother transferred her responsibilities for the care of her five children to her eldest daughter, age 16. The daughter, in turn, quit school, assumed the full caretaker role for her siblings, and became her father's confidante as he watched his wife resign herself to her cancer. The changes imposed on families by illness are limitless and accompanied by a host of feelings: loss, fear, anger, resignation, anxiety, sadness, resentment, and dependency.

How families have coped previously will influence how they negotiate the impact of the illness on their family roles, rules, patterns of communication, and structures. Therefore, in understanding the impact of the illness on the family, some key questions can guide the doctor's inquiry. At what point is the family in the family life cycle (e.g., starting a family, retirement)? Where is each member in the life cycle (e.g., adolescence, middle age)? What are the developmental tasks for each individual and for the family as a whole? How does the illness affect the achievement of these multiple tasks? What kinds of illnesses has the family experienced? What kinds of support have they mobilized in the past to help them cope with illness? Is there currently an established support network? How has the family dealt with illness in the past? Have they responded with functional or dysfunctional patterns of behavior? For example, has the family demonstrated potential maladaptive responses, such as rejection of the sick person, or overprotection that stifles responsibility for self-care?

These latter questions are important because they elicit how families may contribute to or perpetuate illness behavior in their members. The family may represent a safe refuge for the ill person or, conversely, may aggravate the illness through maladaptive responses.

The impact of the diagnosis on the patient and the family will depend on what juncture in the life cycle it occurs. For example, an adult male with a preexisting history of diabetes mellitus may find his disease has less impact on his role (as a husband and father) than does a teenager diagnosed at the point when the family is struggling with adolescent issues of independence and identity. Similarly, the preoccupations and struggles of families in each stage may be vastly different (e.g., how the diagnosis of multiple sclerosis affects the child-rearing responsibilities of the family system; what meaning the death of an adult child has on parents preparing for retirement).

The diagnosis of a debilitating disease affects all family members. One parent (usually the mother) may give up a career to remain home to care for a chronically ill child. For example, the diagnosis of Down's syndrome may force parents into an unexpected role of caregiver beyond the normally expected years of direct parenting or may be perceived by siblings as depleting their parents' availability when the demands of an ill child take precedence. Thus responsibility for care of the sick person may conflict with the needs of other family members.

Finally, although the illness of an individual family member reverberates throughout the family system, the family also plays a powerful role in modifying the illness experience of the individual. A strong body of research now demonstrates how families affect illness in aspects such as the health of husbands and wives (Fisher et al., 1993), mother-infant bonding (Klaus & Kennell, 1976), and the consequences of bereavement (Helsing & Szklo, 1981; Kaprio, Koskenvou, & Rita, 1987). Both McWhinney (1989c) and McDaniel and colleagues (1990) provide excellent reviews of the empirical evidence documenting the significant influence of the family on the health and disease of its members.

Context and Systems

Context includes the disease, the illness, the person, and the environment (see Figure 2.1, Chapter 2). Each person is part of multiple and interlocking systems, including his or her family, ethnic group, peers, social contacts, work and school environments, and religious group. The health care system represents another significant system as the patient interacts with the doctor and other members of the health care team. Relationships and connections with each system may change when the patient becomes ill, and the role assumed by the patient within each of these systems can be altered significantly, depending on the severity of the illness. Also, the nature and quality of these interlocking systems can facilitate or impede how the patient responds to illness.

McWhinney (1989c, p. 92) identified the following cues or behaviors as indicators of potential problems emanating from the patient's context. These cues should alert the doctor to the need to examine contributing contextual factors.

- Frequent attendance with minor illnesses
- Frequent attendance with the same symptoms or with multiple complaints
- Attendance with a symptom that has been present for a long time
- Attendance with a chronic disease that does not appear to have changed
- Incongruity between the patient's distress and the comparatively minor nature of the symptoms
- Failure to recover in the expected time from an illness, injury, or operation
- Failure of reassurance to satisfy the patient for more than a short period
- Frequent visits by a parent with a child with minor problems (the child as a presenting symptom of illness in the parent)

- An adult patient with an accompanying relative
- Inability to make sense of the presenting problem

The following case example illustrates how a patient's illness is influenced dramatically by contextual factors and threatens his self-esteem and ability to fulfill his roles in his family.

CASE EXAMPLE

A 32-year-old male patient presented for the third time in 4 months with knee pain as a result of a basketball injury received 5 months earlier. He complained that his knee continued to cause him extreme discomfort and that he could see no significant improvement. He had discontinued his physiotherapy treatments and now was requesting medication for the pain. Exploration of his current life circumstances revealed that he was at risk of being laid off from his job as a carpet layer—an occupation that clearly exacerbated his symptoms. Because of the threat of layoff, he could not request time off from work and had terminated his physiotherapy because it conflicted with his work schedule. Further inquiry uncovered that he was several months behind in his rent payments and had been served an eviction notice. With few family members or friends in the community, the patient was at a loss about where to locate shelter for his wife and infant son. The perils of unemployment, homelessness, and failure to fulfill adequately his roles as a husband and a father all affected his ability to recover from his knee injury.

Culture

Culture, perhaps more than any other aspect of patients' context, has a profound impact on their health care. How patients conceptualize and interpret their illness is strongly determined by cultural affiliation. Cultural norms and values influence how patients experience illness, seek care, and accept medical interventions (Kleinman et al., 1978). As McWhinney (1989c) noted, cultural differences not only are based on ethnicity but also include subcultural groups defined by age, social class, gender, sexual preference, education, occupation, and religion. For example, although society in general acknowledges the tragedy of AIDS, members of the gay community view it as a living horror.

When cultural differences exist between patient and doctor, the complexity of the interaction can be staggering. Cassell (1991) outlined some of the many ways in which culture can influence health care.

> Culture defines what is meant by masculine or feminine, what clothes are worn, attitudes toward the dying and the sick, mating behavior, the height of chairs and steps, attitudes toward odors and excreta, where typewriters sit and who uses them, bus stops and bedclothes, how the aged and the disabled are treated. These things, mostly invisible to the well, have an enormous impact on the sick and can be a source of untold suffering. They influence the behaviour of others toward the sick person and that of the sick toward themselves. Cultural norms and social rules regulate whether someone can be among others or will be isolated, whether the sick will be considered foul or acceptable, and whether they are to be pitied or censured. (p. 39)

Several cultural features are to be considered for each of the four aspects (disease, illness, person, and context) of the whole person in this model. Although disease is explained by the conventional medical model, it is not immune to the influence of culture. The conventional medical model and the scientific method are both products of Western culture. Thus our cultural "filters" affect how we, as clinicians, understand and manage diseases (Payer, 1988). Just as the approaches to medical practice differ, the venues employed by patients in meeting their health care needs also vary.

Kleinman et al. (1978) described three overlapping sectors of health care: (a) the popular or lay sector, (b) the folk sector, and (c) the professional sector. *Lay care,* influenced by cultural norms and values, consists of self-treatment, family remedies, and advice from friends, neighbors, and colleagues. *Folk care* includes nontraditional healers, shamans, and spiritualists—all powerful and influential figures within their specific cultural groups. Each realm of health care—lay, folk, and professional—has its own unique explanatory model of illness offering explanations of cause, onset, duration, and treatment (Kleinman et al., 1978).

Thus patients' experience of illness will be profoundly influenced by cultural beliefs about "appropriate" illness behavior and models of care. What counts as a symptom of illness and when to consult family members, lay practitioners, healers, or traditional health care professionals are prescribed by culture.

Other factors contributing to variation in health beliefs and practices of different cultural groups are (a) perceptions about illness causation, (b) perspectives on treatment or curing practices, (c) attitudes and expectations of health care facilities and resources deemed most appropriate for the problem, and (d) specific behaviors and reactions to pain and illness sanctioned by the prevailing culture (Schlesinger, 1985).

Culture has a fundamental effect on the psychological development of the person. A move from one culture to another involves major upheaval and loss, which may have serious effects on self-esteem. Such a transition may be compounded by the trauma of torture and the humiliation of refugee status. Language barriers make it even more difficult to articulate needs and to receive support.

There are different cultural responses to transitions in the family life cycle, such as pregnancy, labor, childbirth, and care of the elderly and dying. Cultural differences in family roles and rules may conflict with the expectations of the doctor. In some cultural groups, the sharing of personal and family concerns with an individual outside the family network is prohibited (Germain, 1984).

What strategies can the doctor use to learn more about the patient's culture? It is the doctor's responsibility to attempt to bridge the cultural gap by becoming as familiar as possible with the patient's cultural traditions and beliefs. For example, it may be useful to explain to patients that it would help the doctor, in caring for them, to know more about them, their home situation, and the country from which they came. The doctors can point out that they are not experts in other cultures and that they need patients' help to understand them better. The doctors might ask for tolerance if they say or do something that would be inappropriate in the patients' homeland and encourage patients to inform them so that they do not repeat the same mistake. This disclosure may be difficult for some patients if they are accustomed to viewing doctors as authorities or if their life experiences have socialized them to respond to authority figures with deference, submissiveness, or fear.

It is important to avoid stereotyping people; every culture is complex and diverse. Often, more differences exist among individuals within a particular culture than between the cultures of the patient and the doctor. The most important and relevant information about patients' cultures comes from the patients themselves. They are the experts on what cultural uniqueness means to them.

Conclusion

In his book *The Illness Narratives: Suffering, Healing, and the Human Condition*, Kleinman (1988) painted a poignant and powerful picture of what it is like to live with a chronic illness—in this case, diabetes. But it is the patient herself who is most articulate in describing how her illness and its multiple cardiac complications ravaged her sense of self, significantly altered her relationships with friends and family, and denied her access to the world she savored and enjoyed. This brief quote captures how the illness affected the patient's life—her individual development, her family, and her interactions with the elements that composed her world.

> How was I going to live with this limitation? What a burden I would be on my family and friends. I feared becoming the town invalid. I was terribly guilty. I had felt all along that my illness had interfered with my relationship to my children. I never had enough time to give them. I was more preoccupied with myself than with their problems. I was in the hospital at critical times for them. Now I would be nothing but a burden. As far as my husband goes, the guilt was worse. After the chest pain, I feared having sexual relations. We became celibate. The claudication, the angina, they interfered with the things we loved: long walks in the country, birding, climbing, sports. I had to become self-centered in order to control my condition. I felt like a survivor—all I was good for was hanging on. (p. 33)

Over time, doctors acquire an abundance of information about their patients that goes beyond a catalogue of diseases and treatments. They begin to know them as people with families, friends, jobs, health beliefs, and cultures. In addition, they learn about their patients' struggles with each stage in the life cycle. Knowledge of individual personality development and family life cycle transitions assists doctors in understanding the impact of illness on the negotiation of developmental tasks or transitions in the family system. Information about patients' contexts can provide valuable insights about the barriers or supports that influence care.

Doctors develop an evolving understanding of the social and developmental context in which their patients live their lives. Usually, this information is not gathered in a single encounter as part of a formal social history, but rather is accumulated during many visits that can span many months or years. As patient and doctor share life experiences, this understanding becomes richer and more detailed. With certain patients, such information may help the doctor understand the patients' complex dynamics and idiosyncratic responses to illness or demands for care. Specific aspects of each patient's family dynamics or developmental difficulties may not necessarily be shared with the patient but may guide the doctor in the management and care of the patient. In other instances, facilitating the patients' awareness of the origin of their conflicts or distress may help them make sense of their struggles and pain. Finally, understanding the whole person can deepen the doctor's knowledge of the human condition, especially the nature of suffering and the responses of persons to sickness (Cassell, 1991; Mayeroff, 1972).

LOST DREAMS

Case Illustrating Component 2:
Understanding the Whole Person

Judith Belle Brown

This case illustrates the application and importance of understanding the whole person. It highlights how what initially appeared to be a simple injury was severely complicated by the patient's individual development, her family life, and her environment in general. We observe how failure to understand these key issues aggravated her problems and, finally, how knowledge of her life and experiences provided her with the opportunity to heal.

Lisa, age 18, broke her ankle while playing competitive soccer at school. She was referred to the orthopedic service of the local general hospital, and after investigation, surgery was performed. After her discharge from the hospital, her case was followed by the surgeon in the outpatient orthopedic clinic. The orthopedic consultant thought her response to surgical treatment was unsatisfactory. Lisa had not complied with instructions to exercise in the immediate postoperative period, and her convalescence was compromised by lack of cooperation with the physiotherapist. When confronted by the doctor about her behavior, Lisa became angry and defensive. The doctor, in turn, felt challenged by her hostility, and their tenuous relationship further deteriorated.

As her convalescence progressed, Lisa continued to experience severe pain and discomfort in her ankle. In addition, she complained of profound fatigue and needed an excessive amount of sleep. She also reported symptoms of dizziness, palpitations, abdominal discomfort, nausea, and episodic diarrhea. The orthopedic surgeon, frustrated by her "noncompliance," advised her that these symptoms were not due to postsurgical complications and suggested that she consult her family physician.

After much persuasion by her parents, who were equally confused by her failure to recover, Lisa reluctantly agreed to visit their family doctor. After receiving the laboratory results from Lisa's physical examination, the family physician hypothesized that Lisa's symptoms were manifestations of anxiety. Her resistant behavior and hostile manner were masking her profound feelings of fear and loss of control.

In response to this new understanding of his patient, the doctor expanded his inquiry, asking her about the impact of the injury on her life.

The doctor observed, "It seems that your ankle injury has been very upsetting and frustrating for you, Lisa. How has it changed things in your life?"

Lisa, with her head bowed and clearly tearful, responded, "Oh, I don't know. It's all changed and nobody understands. I just hurt."

"When did the hurt start, Lisa? When did it begin?" the doctor asked.

"I think I've hurt all my life," responded Lisa. "It's all so confusing, and I just want to get better . . . really."

Lisa was encouraged to return on several occasions, and over the course of the next few weeks she began to talk about her life. She described her parents as deeply religious people who had immigrated to this country after World War II. They had left war-torn Europe with few possessions and had experienced much hardship and deprivation in establishing a new life. But, with perseverance, they had built a productive dairy farm and a secure home for their children. Family values endorsed hard work, religious commitment, and solidarity.

Lisa's place in the family was also significant. She was the youngest child of four, having three older brothers. The children were expected to contribute to running the farm and to participate in regular church activities. There also was a strong emphasis on scholastic achievement. All of her brothers, having excelled academically, had left home to pursue professional careers. In contrast, Lisa's academic record was average, and she questioned her ability for further education. Her dreams had focused on her athletic abilities, particularly her aspirations to be a professional skater.

She had devoted exhaustive energy to her skating, training, and competing, and thus had little time to socialize with her peers. Lisa had never dated, and her friendships were limited to her church youth group.

Over a period of several weeks, Lisa developed insight into her problems. She recognized that she had compensated for poor academic achievement and poor socializing skills by investing all of her time, hopes, and aspirations in her skating and that she had become immensely competitive. Now, because of the injury, the one area of her life in which she had invested all of her hopes and expectations for recognition had been destroyed. Her response to this loss was to develop profound anxiety with periods of depression and withdrawal. As she began to grieve her loss, she was able to relinquish her somatic symptoms and renew her efforts for recovery. Furthermore, she came to understand how the strictness of her upbringing determined her patterns of socialization and her relationships with peers and friends and fueled her competitiveness. Knowledge of her role in the family (youngest, female, and only remaining child at home) helped her realize the origin of her current conflictual relationship with her parents. These insights assisted her in gaining an increased awareness of her individual needs and family relationships, resulting in more adaptive interactions with her family members. It also allowed her to shift her priorities and to move forward with the tasks of adolescence.

Lisa's injury had caused a significant upheaval in her life. The pain she felt was not only the pain of an injured ankle; it was also the pain of frustration, sorrow, and regret for the loss of a way of life that met her needs. Only when she was given the opportunity to describe her life was it possible for the doctor to identify the extent of her problem.

Understanding the patient as a whole person allowed the doctor to expand his knowledge and to view Lisa's injury not solely as a biological event but also as one that included social and psychological factors. An increased awareness and appreciation of her family, social network, religious affiliation, academic and athletic pursuits, and developmental issues assisted the doctor in caring for his patient and facilitated Lisa's recovery and growth.

5

The Third Component

Finding Common Ground

JUDITH BELLE BROWN

W. WAYNE WESTON

MOIRA STEWART

B y using a patient-centered approach, doctors can begin to explore and understand patients' ideas, expectations, feelings, and the effects of their illnesses on functioning. By this means, patients' perceptions of their problems are defined. At the same time, by using conventional clinical methods, including history taking, physical examination, and laboratory tests, physicians establish medical definitions of their patients' problems. Throughout this process, an understanding of the whole person, including disease, illness, context, and personhood, evolves. In this chapter, we examine the third interactive component of the patient-centered method: finding common ground.

To reach mutual understanding or to find common ground often requires that two potentially divergent viewpoints be brought together in a reasonable management plan. Once agreement is reached

AUTHORS' NOTE: Parts of this chapter were published previously in *Canadian Family Physician* (1989), 35, 153-157.

on the nature of the problem, the goals and priorities of treatment must be determined: What will be the patient's involvement in the treatment plan? How realistic is the plan in terms of the patient's perceptions of the illness? What are the patient's wishes and ability to cope? Finally, how does each of the parties—patient and doctor—define his or her role in this interaction?

Many authors describe the clinical encounter as a process in which doctor and patient negotiate to define what is important and what should be done (Anstett, 1981; Heaton, 1981; Quill, 1983). Rubin and Brown (as cited in Like & Zyzanski, 1986), for example, defined *negotiation* as the "process whereby two or more parties attempt to settle what each should give and take, or perform and receive, in a transaction between them" (p. 2). The emphasis here is on the potential conflict between the points of view of the doctor and the patient. This perspective is contractual, rather than a true meeting of minds, and is flawed by a simplistic "either/or" stance, rather than a more holistic "both/and" perspective. We prefer to describe this process as a mutual effort of finding common ground between doctor and patient in three key areas: (a) defining the problem, (b) establishing the goals of treatment, and (c) identifying the roles to be assumed by doctor and patient.

In their book *Getting to Yes,* Fisher and Ury (1983) describe two common and erroneous approaches to negotiating differences. The first they call "hard bargaining": Participants are viewed as adversaries, and the goal is victory. This approach generates bad feelings and mistrust. The second approach they call "soft bargaining": The emphasis here is on building and maintaining the relationship, and the goal is agreement. The risk of this approach is a sloppy agreement. Fisher and Ury recommend an alternative, which they call "principled negotiation." Four basic tactics make up this approach:

1. *Separate the people from the problem.* It is better to see the problem as being "out there" and the participants as working together to attack the problem, not each other.

2. *Focus on interests, not positions.* People tend to stake out a position and defend it as if it were personal territory. Often, the underlying interests are forgotten in the battle.

3. *Generate a variety of possibilities before deciding what to do.* Having too much emotional investment in one approach inhibits creativity.

4. *Use objective criteria to judge the solution, rather than pit one personal opinion against another.*

Defining the Problem

It is a universal human characteristic to explain personal experiences in order to give people a sense of having some control by labeling those experiences. Most patients want a "name" for their illness, or at least an explanation of their problem that makes sense to them (Cassell, 1991; Kleinman, 1988; McWhinney, 1989c). Without some agreement about the nature of what is wrong, it is difficult for a doctor and a patient to agree on a plan of management acceptable to both of them. It is not essential for the physician actually to believe that the nature of the problem is as the patient sees it, but the doctor's explanation and recommended treatment must be at least consistent with the patient's point of view and make sense in the patient's world. People may develop quite magical notions of what is happening to them when they become ill. It seems better to them to have an irrational explanation of the problem than no explanation at all. Thus, the quack who offers help will be preferred to the cryptic physician who offers little. Some patients will even blame themselves for the problem, rather than see the illness as simply random or impersonal.

Problems develop when patient and doctor have differing ideas of the cause of the problems. For example:

- A patient says he is disabled by a back problem, and the doctor thinks he is malingering.
- The doctor has diagnosed hypertension, but the patient insists his blood pressure is probably only elevated because he is nervous in the doctor's office and refuses to see it as a problem.
- The parent of a 6-year-old thinks something is seriously wrong because the child has frequent colds: six a year. The doctor thinks that this number is within normal limits and that the parent is overly protective of the child.

We often get into difficulty in defining patients' problems by inappropriate use of the conventional medical model. In using this model, we run a risk of applying improper treatment for problems that do not fit this model. For example, common problems of living may be mislabeled "chronic anxiety disorder" and treated with long-term anxiolytics as if they were some sort of infectious affliction that could be eliminated with chemicals. The analogy to antibiotic use for infections is striking. We need to be reminded of the aphorism: If your only tool is a hammer, you see every problem as a nail.

CASE EXAMPLE

A socially isolated, lonely patient suffered from chronic pain for 20 years, needing his pain to legitimize his disability pension (his only income) and to provide an occasion to sit down with someone who cared about him and his suffering. He long ago accepted this situation as all he could expect. The doctor realized that the pain the patient experienced as physical pain was a metaphor for his intolerable life pain, but the doctor did not inflict this insight on the patient, recognizing that he could not bear it. It was sufficient that the physician's insight allowed her to care more deeply for the patient and to avoid unnecessary investigation to find a disease that was not there. The doctor responded to the patient's cues and followed his lead in discussing his personal life and his feelings. She helped the patient tell his own story at his own pace and avoided the risk of pushing the patient beyond his limits of tolerance.

Defining the Goals

When a doctor and a patient meet, each has expectations and feelings about the encounter; if these are at odds or inappropriate, difficulties may arise. For example:

- The patient has a sore throat and expects to receive penicillin but instead is urged to gargle with salt water.
- The patient is concerned about innocent palpitations but is found to have high blood pressure. The doctor launches into a treatment of the hypertension without explaining to the patient the benign nature of the cardiac symptoms.
- The patient demands muscle relaxants for chronic muscular pains, but the doctor wants to use "talking" therapy to resolve the "underlying" problems.

If doctors ignore their patients' expectations, they risk not understanding their patients, who, in turn, will be angry or hurt by this perceived lack of interest or concern. Some patients will become more demanding in a desperate attempt to be heard; others will become sullen and uncooperative. Patients may be unwilling to listen to their doctors unless they believe they first have been listened to themselves. Hearing fully their patients' distress often challenges doctors to use their imagination and feelings to enter into their patients' inner lives, to experience empathically their patients' pain, confusion, hopes, and fears. This experience may be both threatening and emotionally draining for physicians.

Inexperienced physicians are often uncomfortable with the conventional biomedical responsibility of making the correct diagnosis and are hesitant to add another dimension to a task that already seems difficult enough. Physicians sometimes are concerned that a patient may ask for something they disagree with because they are not comfortable with confrontation and, saying no, they may prefer to avoid an issue. Perhaps they hope the patient will get the message, indirectly, that any ideas not raised by the doctor are unimportant. Students often point out that if they ask patients for ideas and expectations, they will be told, "You're the doctor!" a remark that may leave the students feeling foolish and unable to respond.

Timing is important. If the physician asks for a patient's expectations too early in the interview, the patient may think the doctor is evading making a diagnosis and therefore may be reluctant to say much. If the doctor waits until the end of the interview, however, time may be wasted on issues unimportant to the patient. The physician even may make suggestions that will have to be retracted. Doctors need to express their questions clearly and sincerely. For example, a physician might say, "Can you help me understand what you hope I might do for you today?" It is important that neither the physician's words nor tone of voice suggest any accusation that the patient is wasting the doctor's time on something trivial or silly. Often, it is helpful to pick up on a patient's comments that suggest or hint at his or her ideas, expectations, or feelings—for example, "I have had this chest cold for 3 weeks now, and none of those cough medicines you recommended has helped!"

The doctor should avoid becoming defensive in trying to justify previous advice. Instead, it is more helpful to pick up on the patient's frustration and the implied message that something must be done: "You sound fed up with the length of time this illness has dragged on. Are you wondering if it is something serious? Are you wanting a particular means to clear it up?"

Thus, the goals of treatment must take into account the expectations and feelings of both physician and patient. If the hidden agendas are not recognized, it may be difficult to reach agreement. What physicians call "noncompliance" may be a patient's expression of disagreement about treatment goals; in this sense, the patient always has the last word. The following two examples illustrate some problems in defining goals.

CASE EXAMPLE

Mrs. C. had metastatic breast cancer, and her pain was poorly controlled. Her physician believed that a course of chemotherapy would help. The patient, however, considered this treatment too aggressive and the potential side effects unacceptable. In this case, the physician placed a higher priority on slowing the progress of the disease, whereas the patient wished to concentrate on symptom control.

CASE EXAMPLE

Mrs. Y. was a young mother with three small children. She presented with tennis elbow. The doctor recommended that the patient reduce her activities for several weeks to allow the inflamed area to heal. The patient, however, considered this impossible because of her responsibility for child care. She wanted analgesics to relieve the pain so that she could get on with her jobs.

In these two examples, the physician and the patient needed to work together to find a treatment plan that was acceptable to both. This required that the goals and priorities of each be reexamined. It is often helpful for the doctor to explain the nature of the problem clearly and to outline the pros and cons of different approaches. It is important to acknowledge the patient's concerns first so that the patient is aware that the physician is taking these into account.

Defining the Roles of Patient and Doctor

Sometimes there is profound disagreement about the nature of the problem or the goals and priorities for treatment. When such an impasse occurs, it is important to look at the relationship between patient and doctor and at their perception of each other's roles. (The nature and characteristics of the relationship are dealt with in-depth in Chapter 7; here, we focus on problems in role definition.) Doctors, as in the example of the cancer patient, may see themselves wanting to bring about remission and may expect the patient to assume the role of a passive recipient of treatment. Patients, however, may be seeking a physician who expresses concern and interest in their well-being and who is prepared to treat them in the least invasive manner, viewing them as autonomous individuals with a right to have a voice in deciding among various forms of treatment. This is not such a dilemma for doctors when the various forms of treatment are equally effective, but physicians are understandably concerned when the patient chooses a treatment they consider harmful.

Evolution of the patient-doctor relationship over time allows the doctor to see the same patient with different problems in different settings over a number of years and also to see the patient through the eyes of other family members. The physician's commitment is to "hang in" with the patient to the end. Patients need to know they can count on their doctors to be there when they need them. This ongoing relationship colors everything that happens between them. If there are difficulties in their relationship or differing expectations of their roles, they will have problems in working together effectively. For example:

- The patient is looking for an authority who will tell him or her what is wrong and what to do; the physician, however, wants a more egalitarian relationship in which doctor and patient share decision making.
- The patient longs for a deep and meaningful relationship with a parental figure who will make up for everything the patient's own parent never gave; the doctor wants to be a biomedical scientist who can apply the discoveries of modern medicine to patients' problems.

- The physician enjoys a holistic approach to medicine and wants to get to know patients as people; the patient seeks only technical assistance from the doctor.

Commonly, physicians react in one of two ways to problems in their relationships with patients. First, they tend to blame the patient, who often is characterized as a "crock." This response often is chosen to justify ignoring complaints that are not "legitimate" (organic). Patients can be rejected in a variety of ways: They may be subjected to unnecessary and sometimes dangerous or punitive investigations; they may be given pills instead of time; and they may be referred inappropriately to a variety of specialists. They therefore become dissatisfied with physicians, continue to present numerous unresolving complaints, do not comply with treatment, and switch doctors frequently.

Second, it is common for doctors to blame themselves. They believe they must have done something wrong—that if only they knew more or were more skilled at interviewing or therapy, they could save these people from themselves. The rescue fantasy that led many physicians into medicine is severely tested by these patients. Many physicians take courses to improve their patient management skills, hoping to find "The Answer." Only after repeated failure with a variety of approaches are they able to come to terms with their limitations.

A more effective and satisfying reaction is to realize that the problem is not one-sided. As Pogo said, "We have seen the enemy, and they are us!" On realizing this, physicians can give up their need to be perfect and instead be prepared to do their best, to be "good enough," to be real persons to their patients, rather than needing to find someone to blame for the limitations of medicine.

The Process of Finding Common Ground

We believe that the process of finding common ground begins with the physician clearly describing his or her definition of the problem, management goals, and potential roles in the ensuing care.

Subsequent discussion of each description would proceed with (a) the patient having an opportunity to ask questions and raise concerns or issues; (b) a mutual discussion of these questions, concerns, and issues; and (c) an explicit expression by both patient and physician on their agreement with the problem definition or management goal being discussed. In the event of a lack of agreement between physician and patient, a flexible response by the physician would enhance the finding of common ground.

The final two examples illustrate the key concepts of finding common ground: defining the problems, the goals, and the roles of the patient and the doctor.

CASE EXAMPLE 1

A Demanding Patient

Mrs. A. came to the office after making an urgent phone call demanding a repeat prescription for steroid eyedrops. She had experienced a painful red eye 2 months earlier and had seen an ophthalmologist, by referral, who diagnosed acute iritis and prescribed steroid eyedrops. When similar symptoms recurred a few days previously, she started using the drops again. By the time she was seen, she no longer had any symptoms and her eyes looked normal. She was out of drops and was concerned about a flare-up, as she was leaving for a vacation in Bermuda that afternoon. The resident who saw her had been taught in medical school that family doctors should never prescribe steroid eyedrops and insisted she see an ophthalmologist. He was concerned that the patient's history was vague and was not convinced she had a recurrence of her iritis.

The patient adamantly refused to "waste 2 hours" in emergency and preferred to take her chance without eyedrops if he would not prescribe them. The resident, believing he was in a no-win situation, was furious. On the one hand, if he gave her eyedrops (which he was not even sure she needed) and she had complications, he would feel bad; on the other hand, if he refused, the patient might have a flare-up that would ruin her vacation and perhaps even permanently damage her eye. He feared that this type of "unreasonable" patient was likely to sue him either way. The staff physician who had known the patient for several years realized that she rarely backed down. Even after explaining the doctor's concerns (the uncertain diagnosis and the potential harm of treatment or nontreatment), the patient remained adamant in her request. The doctor decided that, on balance and under these restricted circumstances, the patient's interests would best be served by his being flexible and prescribing the steroid eye-drops. He clearly cautioned her on what symptoms to look for.

CASE EXAMPLE 2

A Case of "Severe" Poison Ivy

Mrs. M., 38 years old, presented to the office with a small patch of poison ivy 3 cm in diameter present for 3 days on her left calf. She was angry with the doctor she had seen the previous day because he had refused to prescribe oral corticosteroids and she stated that the rash had "tripled in size overnight." (His description of the lesion in the medical record stated that the rash was 3 cm in diameter when he had seen it.) She was to play in a golf tournament the next day, wanted to wear shorts, and wanted the rash to be gone; she demanded oral prednisone.

When the doctor explored her concern that the rash might spread, Mrs. M. reported that her son had had a bad case of poison ivy initially treated with topical steroid and then requiring prednisone. She could not be reassured that this was very unlikely to happen in her case, especially after 3 days.

The doctor had known this patient for many years and was aware of her troubled marriage and her great difficulty in trusting anyone. He also knew she often was concerned about her appearance and hated getting older. Experience had taught him that any exploration of these issues was fraught with danger; Mrs. M. would almost certainly become angry and accuse him of not taking her concerns seriously. He decided to focus on her concerns until he was sure she knew he understood and was not taking them lightly. Then he directly addressed their difference of opinion about what was likely to happen and about appropriate management. He asked her to read the adverse effects of prednisone in the *Compendium of Pharmaceuticals and Specialties*. He promised to see her again early the next morning if the rash doubled or tripled in size again and to reconsider oral steroids if that occurred. He made a point of carefully measuring the lesion, telling her its dimensions, and making sure she noticed him recording this in his notes.

Reluctantly, Mrs. M. accepted topical treatment and did not call back. Several months later, when seen for a separate problem, Mrs. M.

mentioned that the poison ivy had become worse the next day but "not too bad."

In both of these cases there was some disagreement about the nature or severity of the problems and appropriate goals or methods of treatment. Also, some difficulties in the patient-doctor relationship could easily have reached an impasse. By being clear in his explanations, by clarifying their differences of opinion while at the same time showing respect for the patient's point of view, and by engaging in a mutual discussion, the physician was able to avoid a harmful power struggle and perhaps sowed the seeds for a more effective working relationship in the future.

In summary, developing an effective management plan requires physicians and patients to reach agreement in three key areas: (a) the nature of the problem, (b) the goals and priorities of treatment, and (c) the roles of the doctor and the patient. Often, doctors and patients have widely divergent views in each of these areas. The process of finding a satisfactory resolution is not so much one of bargaining or negotiating, but rather of moving toward a meeting of minds or finding common ground. This framework reminds physicians to incorporate patients' ideas, feelings, and expectations into treatment planning.

Case Illustrating Component 3:
Finding Common Ground

Martin J. Bass
Judith Belle Brown

Mr. K. arrived at his doctor's office determined that today was the day he would quit smoking. After 30 years of missed starts and failed attempts, he had concluded that the nicotine patch, the latest product on the market, was his answer to success. Several of his friends, also long-term smokers, had endorsed this medication as the reason they had kicked the habit. Thus, without hesitation, Mr. K. insisted that the doctor prescribe this medication immediately.

The doctor, although pleased by her patient's decision, was openly skeptical about such a decision. From her prior experience and from a recent lecture, the doctor knew that patient awareness of triggers to smoking and preparing appropriate distractions were key to smoking cessation. Research also indicated that establishing and preparing for a "quit date" in the near future was an essential aspect of a successful outcome.

Thus the doctor responded by conveying her concerns about the lack of success in using the patch without adequate preparation. She acknowledged the patient's earnest attempt but suggested that he consider these factors (quit date, triggers, distractions) and return to discuss them in 1 week. As the doctor continued to describe the most appropriate methods of smoking cessation, she became aware of Mr. K.'s increasing agitation, cues to his discomfort about the sug-gested management plan. She was somewhat surprised when the patient abruptly concluded the interview with a gruff, "Yeah, Doc, see ya—maybe."

At the end of the day, while completing her charts, the doctor reflected on her encounter with Mr. K. The patient had indicated he wanted help to quit smoking; the doctor had offered her expert advice, but the visit had ended unsatisfactorily for both the patient and the doctor. The doctor pondered the following questions: What had gone wrong during the visit? Why had Mr. K. become angry? How could she change future interactions to circumvent similar patient reactions? Had she, the doctor, missed something pertinent that resulted in the patient's hostile response?

The patient's anger and apparent dissatisfaction with his doctor may be understood from several perspectives. For the patient, this was "the critical moment" when he had decided to quit smoking. In his mind, he had a clear plan of action of how this goal could be achieved. He had not been prepared for the doctor's detailed description of the protocol required for successful smoking cessation. Because the patient expected the doctor to be pleased by his decision to quit smoking, he had not anticipated the doctor's cautionary tone. Nor had he expected the doctor's reticence to prescribe the medication without proper preparation. The patient had become angry because his expectations of the visit had not been met. The patient and the doctor had not shared the same perceptions of the problem or a common understanding of the treatment plan.

From the doctor's perspective, her management of the problem had been based on empirical evidence and sound clinical judgment. Her approach to the problem and plans for addressing the patient's decision to quit smoking were not in error. Absent in the encounter was an attempt by the doctor to elicit the patient's opinion of the doctor's suggested plan of action in a spirit of partnership. This effort might have reinforced the doctor's understanding of the patient's expressed need "to quit now." For example, missing the patient's readiness to tackle this addiction here and now might have been avoided by (a) pauses during the doctor's description of the management, allowing time for patient questions and reactions; (b) encouragement by the doctor of a mutual discussion on the matter; and (c) explicit checking of the patient's agreement on the plan.

As the doctor reviewed her discussion with Mr. K., she realized that she had not come to a mutual understanding and agreement of what treatment approach would be most acceptable and viable for her patient. Although she believed in following his protocol for smoking cessation, she also acknowledged that one must listen to the patient's ideas about a management plan and begin where the patient is. Only then would a common understanding be established that would promote successful treatment. The doctor decided that perhaps next time, if a similar request was made, she immediately would enter into a two-way discussion with a view to establishing a partnership leading to agreement.

One week later, Mr. K. surprisingly returned with the news that 2 weeks hence he would quit smoking. The doctor reinforced her patient's decision and, without reservation, prescribed the nicotine patch. In addition, and most important, she acknowledged her lack of attending to the patient's initial request. This disclosure gave the doctor and the patient an opportunity to discuss how they might achieve common ground more readily in the future.

NOTE: This case description first appeared in the January 1993 issue of the *Ontario Medical Review* and is reprinted with the permission of the Ontario Medical Association.

6

The Fourth Component

Incorporating Prevention and Health Promotion

CAROL L. MCWILLIAM

THOMAS R. FREEMAN

All health professionals currently are challenged to promote health, as well as to prevent disease. The patient-centered approach allows professionals to maximize their contributions to these health care activities because health, like disease and illness, requires an integrated understanding of the whole person. Furthermore, disease prevention and health promotion require a collaborative effort on the part of patient and physician, who therefore must find a common ground in order for these activities to be pursued. This chapter builds on the preceding three chapters to illustrate how the patient-centered approach facilitates focus on health promotion and disease prevention and, in turn, how focus on prevention and health promotion incorporates the patient-centered approach.

The Foundations of
Health Promotion and Disease Prevention

In 1984, the World Health Organization (WHO, 1986b) redefined *health* as "a resource for everyday life, not the objective of living. This concept of health emphasizes social and personal resources as well as physical capacities" (p. 73). Thus, the notion of health is moving away from its former abstract focus on complete physical, mental, and social well-being toward an ecological understanding of the interaction between individuals and their social and physical environment (de Leeuw, 1989; Hurowitz, 1993; Stachtchenko & Jenicek, 1990). How patients and practitioners think about and experience health continues to evolve. Therefore, these partners in health care have unique and often differing understandings of health and, in turn, different understandings of health promotion and disease prevention. Applying the patient-centered approach is essential to understanding this element of the context of care.

The process of care also has been altered and continues to evolve in the light of new definitions. *Health promotion* most recently has been defined (WHO, 1986a) as "the process of enabling people to take control over and to improve their health" (p. 73). The intervention strategy for promoting health has been labeled "health enhancement"—or increasing the level of good health, vitality, and resilience in all people.

Unlike health promotion, *disease prevention* is aimed at reducing the risk of acquiring a disease. As a process, disease prevention reduces the likelihood that a disease or disorder will affect an individual (Stachtchenko & Jenicek, 1990). Disease prevention strategies fall into three familiar categories: (a) risk avoidance, (b) risk reduction, and (c) early identification. *Risk avoidance* aims at ensuring that people at low risk for health problems remain at low risk by finding ways to avoid disease. *Risk reduction* addresses moderate- or high-risk characteristics among individuals or segments of the population by finding ways to cure or control the prevalence of disease. *Early identification* aims at increasing the awareness of early signs of health problems and screening people at risk in order to detect the early onset of health problems.

Whether the process of health care is to be health enhancement, risk avoidance, risk reduction, or early identification of disease depends on the relationship between the timing of the opportunity for intervention and the patient's potential for disease at that time. Most important, both preventive care and health promotion efforts depend on the patient's state of health and commitment to the pursuit of health. Thus, the patient-centered approach is also essential to the process of promoting health and preventing disease. As described in the preceding chapters, effective patient care requires attending to the patients' personal experience of health, illness, and disease; understanding patients in the context of their lives; and finding commonly agreed-on approaches to preventive care and health promotion.

Health Promotion and
Disease Prevention Requires Patient-Centered Care

The importance of the patient-centered approach to achieving health promotion and disease prevention must not be underestimated. Health promotion and disease prevention are important pillars in the "new public health movement" as described in the Ottawa Charter (Epp, 1986). Much of the energy directed toward these thrusts has been devoted to developing public policy, screening, and other methods and to addressing related ethical issues (Doxiadis, 1987; Hoffmaster, 1992). Almost all involved have taken a population-based approach to health. With notable exceptions (Audunsson, 1986; McWilliam, 1993), little attention has been paid to implementing ideas of health promotion and disease prevention at the level of the individual practitioner and client/patient. Yet, achieving new directions clearly hinges on individual, as well as collective, effort. The patient-centered clinical method provides a clear framework for the practitioner to apply in health promotion and disease prevention efforts by using the patient's world as the starting point.

UNDERSTANDING THE PATIENT'S WORLD

A patient-centered approach to health promotion and disease prevention begins with an understanding of the whole person in context (Weston et al., 1989). To achieve such an understanding, the physician must assess five components of the patient's world: (a) present and potential disease, (b) the patient's experience of health and illness, (c) the patient's potential for health, (d) the patient's context, and (e) the patient-doctor relationship.

Present and Potential Disease. In Chapter 2, Weston and Brown define disease as "a theoretical construct, or abstraction, by which physicians attempt to explain patients' problems in terms of abnormalities of structure and/or function of body organs and systems and includes both physical and mental disorders." Human existence, by its very nature, carries with it the presence of the individual's potential or declared disease status. Each patient's world, therefore, invites the tradition of health enhancement, risk avoidance, risk reduction, or early identification of disease. In keeping with concern about human potential for disease, much of the literature in primary care pertaining to prevention deals with appropriate screening maneuvers (Canadian Task Force on the Periodic Health Examination, 1979; U.S. Preventive Services Task Force, 1989) and establishing a practice infrastructure to bring these about (Audunsson, 1986; Battista & Lawrence, 1988).

The Patient's Experience of Health and Illness. To understand the perspective of the patient, the practitioner needs to explore the patient's beliefs in relation to health and illness and what each means to that person (Calnan, 1988). The practitioner needs to discover the value and priority of health as one of many competing values in order to assess the patient's commitment to its pursuit. Fundamental to determining common ground regarding preventive behavior is the extent to which the individual feels responsible for and in control of his or her own health. Beliefs about health risks and the degree of control a patient has over those risks will affect his or her actions.

The patient's experience of health and illness subsumes the patient's ideas about susceptibility, seriousness, benefits, and barriers that are experienced as feelings, expectations, and ways of functioning (Weston et al., 1989). Researchers have found a significant positive correlation between self-reported perceived health status and a health-promoting lifestyle (Gillis, 1993). In addition, studies have identified that individuals who conceive of health as the presence of wellness, rather than as merely the absence of disease, have a significantly stronger engagement in health-promoting lifestyles (Gillis, 1993). Thus, it is important to assess both the patient's own perception of experienced health and illness and what health really means in daily life.

Perceived benefits and barriers to health and health-promoting lifestyles are equally important. Several studies have identified that potential strategies for promoting health are adopted only if they are perceived to be beneficial. Likewise, others have found that the greater the individual's perceptions of barriers to health, the lower that person's health status (Gillis, 1993).

In summary, the more illness-oriented a patient's experience, the more the patient's world calls for the doctor to act as healer or therapeutic interventionist. If the patient perceives little seriousness or susceptibility to illness and great benefits to health promotion and prevention, the patient's world calls for the doctor to be a facilitator and educator. Likewise, the less fear and embarrassment experienced in the role of patient and the greater the self-confidence and self-direction of the patient, the more appropriate is the practitioner's role as facilitator and educator.

The Patient's Potential for Health. The patient's potential for health is determined by age, gender, genetic potential for disease, socioeconomic status, and personal goals and values. Perhaps the most challenging component of assessing a patient's potential for health lies in identifying personal goals and values. The patient's valuing of health cannot be assumed. Yet, holding this value is logically fundamental to a health-promoting lifestyle, and a positive correlation between the two has been demonstrated in many studies (e.g., Gillis, 1993).

Self-efficacy—the power to produce one's own desired ends—is fundamental to the patient's potential for health. Bandura (1986) suggested that self-efficacy behavior, which includes choice, effort, and persistence in activities related to desired goals or outcomes, is a function of (a) the individual's self-perceptions of ability to perform a behavior and (b) the individual's beliefs that the behavior in question will lead to the specific outcomes desired. Numerous studies document the positive correlation between these two factors and actual decision making regarding health behavior (Brod & Hall, 1984; Ewart, Taylor, Reese, & DeBusk, 1983; Jeffrey et al., 1984; Jenkins, 1987; Kaplan, Atkins, & Reinsch, 1984; McIntyre, Lichtenstein, & Mermelstein, 1983; Nicki, Remington, & MacDonald, 1984). Although research related to the influence of locus of control is contradictory, researchers have demonstrated that self-efficacy and health status are the most powerful predictors of a health-promoting lifestyle (Gillis, 1993).

To summarize, the more favorable the patient's potential for health, particularly as it relates to self-efficacy and health status, the more appropriate the practitioner's role as facilitator of health enhancement and as educator regarding risk avoidance. The less favorable the patient's potential for health, the more appropriate the doctor's intervention with risk reduction and early identification strategies.

The Patient's Context. The patient's context, the physical and interpersonal environment of the person, includes family, friends, job, community, and culture (Epp, 1986; Watson, 1984). Mass media can influence health attitudes and beliefs in both subtle and obvious ways and may either enhance the patient's potential for health or detract from it (National Research Council, 1989). Similarly, the availability or absence of such resources as social support groups may enhance or detract from the individual's potential for health.

Likewise, the doctor's office setting is an important part of the patient's context. The "personal" element and emphasis on continuity of care may make the family physician's office setting more conducive than other medical settings to the type of patient-doctor relationship necessary for the practice of health education (Calnan, 1988). Yet, family doctors have found that lack of time, space, and necessary staff are barriers to preventive activities (Becker & Janz, 1990; Bruce & Burnett, 1991; Pommerenke & Dietrich, 1992). Office hours, location, and physical structure have the potential to represent real barriers from the patient's perspective. Ease of access, proximity to such screening resources as mammography sites, and the privacy and comfort of the doctor's office all constitute contextual factors that influence the patient's receptivity to using the family physician as a resource for health promotion and disease prevention (Carter, Belcher, & Inui, 1981; Godkin & Catlin, 1984). Furthermore, the skills, perceptions, and attitudes of office staff, particularly the office nurse, affect patients. Staff need to be supportive of the doctor's health promotion and disease prevention efforts by providing positive reinforcement to patients, especially reinforcing patients' perceptions that changing health-related behavior is possible.

To summarize, the patient's context is an essential component of any effort to promote health or to prevent disease. A supportive social context is particularly important for successful health enhancement. The doctor's office context can be designed intentionally to enhance all strategies to promote health and to prevent disease.

The Patient-Doctor Relationship. Very much a part of the patient's context and potential for health is the nature of the patient's relationship with the doctor and personal experience of care. Built over time, the physician's approach determines how much and what kind of trust the patient places in the physician, what the patient's expectations of the roles of doctor and patient are, and what kind of power relationship exists between them (Brody, 1992). The patient's approach to assuming or relinquishing power to the physician shapes the physician's approach to patient care and, ultimately, the patient-doctor relationship. Thus, the doctor's power to intervene both shapes and is shaped by the patient's world.

Investigation of the impact of the patient-doctor relationship on health promotion and disease prevention has been limited. Nevertheless, several authors (Pommerenke & Dietrich, 1992; Quill, 1989; Sanson-Fisher & Maguire, 1980) have noted that poor physician communication skills may be one of the most important and overlooked barriers to preventive care.

In summary, health promotion and disease prevention require a patient-centered approach. Knowledge of the patient's present and potential disease, the patient's experience of both health and illness, and the patient's experience of the context of health and health care facilitates the choice, implementation, and success of health promotion and disease prevention strategies. The physician's patient-centeredness ensures greater success in promoting health and preventing disease.

Patient-Centeredness Facilitates
Health Promotion and Disease Prevention

Applying the patient-centered approach allows the practitioner to find the methods of health promotion and preventive care that most appropriately match the patient's world. The patient's world may be viewed as an integrated system, and the components of this system together create a whole that is different from the sum of the parts. The practitioner's knowledge of this world helps in making a judgment about which health promotion or disease prevention strategy provides the most appropriate fit.

The doctor and the patient together find common ground (Brown, Weston, & Stewart, 1989), arriving at decisions about the goals and priorities of care and their respective roles in it. If the most recent definitions of health care are to be enacted, strategy selection in health

promotion and disease prevention calls for special attention to appropriately sharing power. Being alert to the sense of powerlessness that
patients often experience, supporting and encouraging the patient's
own exercise of power "so long as it is consistent with a good therapeutic outcome and with the patient's long-term goals and interests"
(Brody, 1992, p. 65), and using "the physician-patient relationship as
a primary therapeutic tool" (p. 65) are all a part of the process of
finding common ground. Through this process, the physician and the
patient together decide the health promotion and prevention strategies to be pursued.

Strategy selection within the patient-centered model also requires
the doctor to adopt current thinking about adult learning and to
approach health promotion with adult patients accordingly. The
patient-centered educational approach in health promotion is a
learner-centered social process (see Chapter 11). The doctor precipi-
tates the patient-learner's critical reflection about health through
dialogue that makes the patient aware of the potential threats to health
inherent in the individual's current life. The physician guides the
patient through exploration of the personal meaning of current practices and the personal values, needs, motives, expectations, and understandings that underlie these life elements. Over time, the process
of guiding the patient-learner also includes exploring alternative
ways of looking at current practices and of finding and trying new
ways of fulfilling personal values, needs, motives, and expectations.
A supportive role is also part of this process: listening, empathizing,
validating changed perspectives through rational discourse, and
working out new relationships with the patient-learner, consistent
with changes in perspective.

The learning is self-discovered and cannot be communicated directly by the physician; rather, the physician is guided by the conditions of learning (Rogers, 1961). The commonly known strategies of
health education, most of which emphasize information giving and
behavior modification, comprise only a small part of the process of
health promotion. For true personal growth and change to transpire,
the patient-centered approach is critical.

The patient's world is understood as a dynamic situation that varies
with each patient at different points in time and with each health care
issue. The doctor's aim is to find the best fit with the patient's world.
Sometimes, for some issues, the patient requires a health enhancement
strategy. At other times, for other reasons, the patient requires preven-

tion strategies. The following examples illustrate how the doctor uses the patient-centered approach in choosing and implementing a strategy for health promotion and/or disease prevention.

CASE EXAMPLE 1

George K., a 35-year-old insurance adjuster, had been found to have blood pressures between 130-135/90-95 during three successive visits. He had smoked a pack of cigarettes a day for the past 15 years and had consumed 8 to 10 bottles of beer a week, usually on weekends. He also had led a sedentary life. Recently, George's father underwent coronary bypass surgery at the age of 64, having had symptoms of angina for about 5 years. George had never taken much interest in his health until his recent marriage. Generally, he had viewed physicians with some suspicion, but his current family physician had earned his respect when she attended him after his appendectomy 5 years ago.

When George presented at the office, the doctor used a preventive medicine model, screening him for other risk factors of heart disease and end-organ damage. Being patient-centered, she recognized that the new marriage could play a significant role in motivating George to a healthier lifestyle and that George's new wife could be included in health teaching regarding diet and exercise. Capitalizing on George's receptivity to health teaching and newly acquired social support, she also addressed the need to quit smoking, exercise more regularly, and optimize weight.

CASE EXAMPLE 2

Sandra B. was 16 years old. While in the doctor's office for her monthly allergy shot, she noticed a waiting room poster designed to draw attention to the disadvantages of unplanned pregnancy. She had been dating another student in her high school and was aware that their relationship soon may involve sexual intercourse. Sandra had been in good health all her life and, because of her interest in sports and physical fitness, took the maintenance of her health very seriously. She was aware of the importance of a balanced diet and regular exercise. She had been going to her current family doctor since her childhood and was generally on good terms with him. Approaching him regarding the birth control pill, however, raised fears that her parents eventually would find out because they also have attended the same doctor. Sandra therefore decided to make an appointment for knee pains that had been bothering her. If doing so seemed safe enough, she intended to bring up the issue of birth control on the same visit.

When Sandra presented in the office, the patient-doctor relationship was tested in the crucible of adolescence. Using a patient-centered approach, the physician maintained a nonjudgmental attitude and openness to discussing Sandra's concerns and thereby facilitated Sandra's verbalization of her wishes. Acting as health educator, the physician provided information about birth control, as well as prevention of sexually transmitted disease. Using health enhancement strategies, he also explored with Sandra the psychosocial aspects of sexual behavior. Subsequent visits emphasized the need for regular screening procedures, such as pap smears, once she became sexually active. The encounter served to empower this young woman with respect to her health and gave her a sense of self-worth and heightened self-esteem.

CASE EXAMPLE 3

Barbara H. was 48 years old when she attended her family physician for a routine examination. She was very concerned that her menstrual periods had been irregular in the past year. Having read about menopause in magazines and newspapers, Barbara had a number of questions about hormone replacement therapy (HRT). She feared increased risk of cancer but had heard that HRT may prevent osteoporosis. She recalled that her mother had suffered from several broken bones and had a stooped posture for years prior to her death of breast cancer at the age of 78.

Barbara had no significant health problems. She had three children, born in her late 20s and early 30s. All had been breast fed. Barbara had attended her family physician on a regular basis for a number of years, and checkups had been fine. All pap smears had been normal. Barbara recently had begun to pay more attention to her health, as the children had grown and no longer needed so much attention from her. She had joined an exercise class and had begun to take tennis lessons. Her marriage was stable, and she worked outside the home as a legal secretary on a part-time basis.

Barbara always had expected her physician to take the lead in recommending advice about her health. She was comfortable with this and has had a trusting relationship with him.

Using a health education approach, Barbara's physician explained to her the known risks and benefits of HRT. Employing health enhancement strategies, together they considered how current recommendations (American College of Physicians, 1992) may or may not be applicable in her particular case. Barbara's physician was concerned about the history of breast cancer in a first-degree relative, but this history had to be weighed against the risk of the development of osteoporosis and coronary disease. After due discussion, patient and doctor together decided to emphasize optimal nutrition and exercise for the present time. They also agreed that, at a later date, they may elect to use bone densitometry to ascertain whether she is at increased risk for osteoporosis. In addition, Barbara's physician took this opportunity to underline the importance of regular breast examination and, at a later date, mammographic screening.

The strategies that physicians employ will vary from patient to patient and from time to time with the same patient, depending on the circumstances, the life stage of the patient, and the presence or absence of health-risk behavior. Deciding on an appropriate strategy ultimately means finding common ground. Of course, no strategy is pursued without the patient's informed consent (Lee, 1993).

Achieving informed consent presents a particular challenge in the areas of health promotion and disease prevention. Because the benefits or risks of a preventive procedure generally are determined on societal, rather than an individual, level, it is not possible to predict the consequences for any one person (Hanckel, 1984). The tendency has been to weigh the benefits and potential harm of a preventive procedure such as immunization on a societal, rather than an individual, level (Rose, 1981). However, the physician has a moral and ethical responsibility to present to the patient the risks and psychological costs of proposed prevention programs (Marteau, 1990). In addition, it must be made clear that the problems are difficult to predict in advance and that little is known about the prognosticators of health (Schoenbach, Wagner, & Karon, 1983). Even when problems and prognosticators are predicted correctly, known treatments only work for a portion of patients, and that portion cannot be identified. Thus, physicians cannot tell a patient how certain they might be that the preventive treatment will produce the desired effect (Hanckel, 1984).

Clearly, health promotion and disease prevention necessitate increased physician effort to address the ethical issues of care (Strasser, Jeanneret, & Raymond, 1987). Ultimately, patients have the right to choose and, in so choosing, share the responsibility for outcomes. This, too, is an important parameter of health, health promotion, and disease prevention.

Conclusion

Evidence is compelling that health promotion and prevention efforts can be applied effectively by physicians. Yet, both physician education and attitudes (McPhee, Richard, & Solkowit, 1986; McPhee & Schroeder, 1987) and patient education, expectations, motivations, and attitudes (McGinnis & Hamburg, 1988) can undermine such interventions. Overcoming such barriers to achieve success in health promotion and disease prevention efforts can be achieved by using a patient-centered approach.

"AN OUNCE OF PREVENTION . . .
A POUND OF CURE"

First Case Illustrating Component 4:
Incorporating Prevention
and Health Promotion

Thomas R. Freeman
Moira Stewart
Judith Belle Brown

Mrs. B.: Doctor, my husband and I thought about having Jason vaccinated, but after reading some books, we're not so sure it's the right thing to do.

Doctor: Tell me about your concerns.

The B.s, responsible and conscientious parents of 6-month-old Jason, were new to their family doctor's practice. The doctor was surprised to find that the child had received no vaccinations.

A bright and well-educated couple, Mr. and Mrs. B. had taken time to inform themselves on infant and baby care. The B.s had invested in a good-quality baby car seat and were very interested in planning for the baby's future, yet they were reluctant to have Jason immunized. They had been aware of sensational media reports of presumed vaccine adverse effects resulting in permanent neurological damage. These reports had left them doubtful about the benefits and risks of vaccination for their son.

In contrast, their family physician saw vaccination as a basic investment in Jason's future health. It may be difficult for a physician to understand a patient's opposing viewpoint, given the clear benefits made possible by vaccination programs (Koplan, Schoenbeum, Weinstein, & Fraser, 1979). For many reasons, the lay public may evaluate medical risks differently from the "experts." Research in the field of decision making has found that people's perceptions of risk are not determined by rational processes, but rather that greater weight is given to risks if the risk is perceived to be involuntary, is dreaded, is immediate, appears to be uncontrollable, puts children at risk, or is unfamiliar (Whyte & Burton, 1982).

Media attention has played a significant role in shaping the public's perception of vaccinations. In some countries, such attention has been instrumental in the decline in vaccination rates and the resultant resurgence of previously controlled infectious diseases (Cherry, 1984). Perceived risk has been found to be one variable in a person's decision about whether or not to participate in a program of disease prevention (Adjaye, 1981; Carter & Jones, 1985; Morgan, Lakhani, Morris, & Vaile, 1987).

The B. family had serious reservations about allowing vaccination of their child. Their family physician listened carefully to their concerns and answered them respectfully. She put the small risks of vaccine side effects into perspective by comparing the published risks of adverse vaccine reactions with the risks of everyday events. For example, the risk of encephalopathy following measles vaccination is less than 1 in 1 million, which compares very favorably with the 1 in 2,000 risk of encephalopathy in those who actually get measles. Other activities that increase the chance of death by 1 in 1 million are smoking 1.4 cigarettes, living 2 months with a smoker, traveling 30 miles by car, and flying 1,000 miles by jet (British Medical Association, 1987).

After careful consideration of these points, Mr. and Mrs. B. decided to have their son Jason immunized; this was done without any side effects.

In this case, the family physician found common ground with the parents and came to a mutually satisfactory agreement by recognizing that it is possible to have legitimate opinions that differ from the "experts" and then by listening carefully to the concerns raised by those opinions and addressing those concerns in a forthright manner.

NOTE: This case description first appeared in the October 1991 issue of the *Ontario Medical Review* and is reprinted with the permission of the Ontario Medical Association.

CHOICES AND CHANCES—
WHOSE RESPONSIBILITY?

Second Case Illustrating Component 4:
Incorporating Prevention and Health Promotion

Carol L. McWilliam
Judith Belle Brown

When you're 80 years old and you're longing for something, I don't think one or two cigarettes would hurt you. I would never let anybody want so much for something! I've been pretty good these days—not too much trouble breathing. Doctors and nurses have what they want! They smoke when they want. But their day is coming! They should realize I haven't got anything else in life. What the heck am I living for?

Mrs. Q. clearly was frustrated and disillusioned with her doctor's "no smoking" order. His expectations that she quit smoking seemed highly unfair. For her, smoking was one of the few pleasures left in life. Every week, she would visit her disabled husband in the nursing home, and, over a cigarette, they would quietly chat, reminiscing about the past. For her, to give up smoking meant forfeiting a meaningful event in her one remaining significant relationship. She knew the risks but was prepared to take the chance.

However, to Dr. S., her family physician, the problem of her smoking was of great concern. The combination of chronic obstructive pulmonary disease and episodes of asthma required absolute restriction of smoking. Another concern was Mrs. Q.'s requirement for occasional home oxygen therapy and the safety hazards that her smoking habits created. Dr. S. was frustrated with Mrs. Q.'s noncompliant behavior and could not understand her failure to accept his preventive treatment protocol. He had outlined clearly the risks and expected her to make reasonable choices.

Who is responsible for these chances and choices? The physician had identified the medical problems and priorities and clearly outlined the direction to be followed. However, the patient's goals and expectations differed significantly from those of her physician. The consequences of the dissonant views of the patient's illness have been noncompliance, dissatisfaction, and criticism of health professionals.

Preventive health care requires moving from traditional notions of patient compliance to viewing patients as autonomous individuals with a right to have a voice in deciding among various approaches to treatment and lifestyle choices. Physicians must be continuously aware of the importance of patients' autonomy and right to self-determiation. In addition, they need to understand social, psychological, and cultural issues that influence cooperation of patients in their care.

In fact, for optimal health promotion to occur, the physician must work collaboratively with patients to empower them to take an active role in planning and managing their own care (McWilliam, 1993). The physician needs to elicit the patients' ideas about their problems, their preferences for treatment, and their understanding of the responsibilities of both the doctor and the patient in management of care. This may necessitate addressing differences of opinion with patients so that together the doctor and the patient may reach a conclusion that is both acceptable and safe for the patient. Finally, the doctor must know when to "give in gracefully" to patients. This requires due consideration of each patient's larger life context.

Health promotion requires sharing responsibility. To achieve mutual agreement and commitment to a reasonable treatment protocol, the doctor must go beyond what appears to be medically prudent or correct and take into consideration the patient's ideas and views. Decisions about choices and changes must consider the patient's life, values, expectations, and priorities.

Returning to Mrs. Q., Dr. S. confronted their differences of opinion, taking into greater consideration her age, life circumstances (sharing life with a dying husband), and meager pleasures in life. Together, they negotiated a plan satisfactory to both. The plan ensured patient safety, encompassed the patient's ability to judge the extent of her breathing problems at any particular point in time, and allowed her to choose to take a few chances in judicious occasional smoking. Choices and chances thereby became a shared responsibility in promoting health.

NOTE: This case description first appeared in the February 1994 issue of the *Ontario Medical Review* and is reprinted with the permission of the Ontario Medical Association.

7

The Fifth Component

Enhancing the Patient-Doctor Relationship

MOIRA STEWART

JUDITH BELLE BROWN

IAN R. McWHINNEY

The relationship is the bedrock or the basis for all interchanges between two people and could be described as a primal exchange between the two individuals. Relationships, in general, involve caring, feeling, trust, power, and a sense of purpose. In a patient-doctor relationship, the purpose is to help the patient (to be a therapeutic relationship and, frequently, to foster healing).

Complex interactions occur between the patient-doctor relationship and the other components of patient-centered communication. For this reason, we frequently allude to material from previous chapters. We divide the chapter into six sections, each covering some well-known conceptualizations of helping relationships. The sections deal with attributes of a therapeutic relationship, power in the patient-doctor relationship, caring, healing, self-awareness, and transference and countertransference.

AUTHORS' NOTE: The authors thank Oxford University Press for permission to quote from E. J. Cassell (1991), *The nature of suffering and the goals of medicine*.

Attributes of a Therapeutic Relationship

)(Many authors, representing various disciplines, have described specific facilitative attributes of the clinician that promote the development and maintenance of the helping relationship. These include empathy, congruence, genuineness, respect, positive regard, and caring and concern for the other (Carkhuff, 1987; Cournoyer, 1991; Dubovsky, 1981; Perlman, 1979; Rogers, 1961). In addition to these core therapeutic qualities are the appreciation of the importance of mutual trust and a readiness to share power and to accept difference (Brody, 1992; Kleinman, 1988; Perlman, 1979; Sherwin, 1992).

Trust lays the groundwork for the possibility of reciprocity. Cassell (1991) highlighted the role of trust and reciprocity in the patient-doctor relationship:

> Doctors are people who, because of their special knowledge, are empowered to act by virtue of the trust given by patients, and who acquire responsibility thereby. In their actions on behalf of the sick person, endangered by the possibility of failing their responsibility, doctors become threatened by what threatens the patient. *Doctor and patient are bound in a reciprocal relationship*—failure to understand that is failure to comprehend clinical medicine. (p. 76)

On the other hand, the relationship is not always reciprocal. Despite this, it remains the doctor's responsibility to be constant in his or her commitment to the well-being of the patient. As Stephens (1982) explained, "Physicians do not have the luxury of limiting their involvement to those patients who can make and keep promises" (p. 164). The required commitment is not achieved easily because the doctor may experience feelings of failure and have to encounter a patient's anger or other expressions of mistrust. Cassell (1991) described constancy in the following way:

> Constancy to the patient is necessary. Constant attention and maintained presence are not difficult when things are going well. It requires self-discipline to maintain constancy when the case is going sour, when errors or failures have occurred, when the wrong diagnosis has been made, when the patient's personality or behavior is difficult or even repulsive, when impending death brings the danger of sorrow and loss

because emotional closeness has been established. When constancy is absent or falters too frequently, patients lose that newfound part of themselves—the doctor—that promised stability in the uncertain world of sickness arising from their relationship. (p. 78)

Power in the Patient-Doctor Relationship

In the literature of the past 20 years, much has been made of power and control in the patient-doctor relationship. The relationship that is the foundation for patient-centered care, compared with the traditional relationship, demands a sharing of power and control between the doctor and the patient (Brody, 1992). Other authors who have proposed models of doctor-patient relationships have variously described the state of high patient control of decision making as mutuality (Szasz & Hollender, 1956), the contractual relationship (Veatch, 1972), and the consumerist approach (Haug & Lavin, 1983; Roter & Hall, 1992; Stewart & Roter, 1989).

These approaches are similar, but not identical, to Component 3, Finding Common Ground, described in Chapter 5 of this book. The quality of a relationship within which finding common ground is possible includes a readiness of doctor and patient to become partners in care. Their encounters are truly meetings between experts (Tuckett, Boulton, Olson, & Williams, 1985). Each partnership is unique and may include permutations and combinations employing varying degrees of control along many dimensions and changing over time. One example is the adolescent who needs information (from the expert doctor) but who also maintains control of management (envisioning herself as the expert on her life) because she yearns to be treated as an adult but at the same time needs guidance. An ability on the part of the doctor to remain open and alert to these shifting needs for control is an essential aspect of a partnership.

The resulting therapeutic alliance is related in complex ways to enhancing patients' sense of self-efficacy—that is, sense of control over themselves and their world or, to put it another way, a sense of omnipotence. We see later in this chapter that these desired outcomes are considered key dimensions of health and wholeness (Cassell, 1991).

Caring

Caring implies that the doctor is fully present and engaged with the patient. The notion of the detached clinician who keeps a safe emotional distance is replaced by the notion that doctor and patient are interconnected in such a deep way that the doctor can be fully immersed in the concerns of the patient (Montgomery, 1993). Intense caring moments in relationships involve mutual recognition on the part of patient and practitioner and a reciprocal learning of both individuals (Frank, 1991; Suchman & Matthews, 1988; Watson, 1985). Boundaries may be much more blurred than in the traditional, distanced, one-way relationship. However, the closeness restores the patient's sense of connectedness (Belenky, Clinchy, Goldberger, & Tarule, 1986; Candib, 1988; Cassell, 1991) to the human race, a connectedness that may have been broken by their physical or emotional suffering.

Frank (1991) said that care is a matter of recognizing that every patient is different: "The common diagnostic categories into which medicine places its patients are relevant to disease, not to illness. They are useful for treatment, but they only get in the way of care" (p. 45). The problem, said Frank, is that most people who deal with ill persons do not want to recognize differences and particularities because to do so takes time and involvement.

For generations, medical students have been taught: "Don't get involved." In the conventional clinical method, the doctor is assumed to be a detached observer and prescriber of treatment. Remaining uninvolved may protect doctors from some very disturbing things, especially in the encounter with suffering. But it also has a personal price. To remain uninvolved, physicians have to build up protective shells to suppress their feelings. This lack of openness makes for difficulties in relationships, not only with patients but also with colleagues. To suggest that one can remain uninvolved is also a fallacy. One cannot help being affected in some way by the encounter with suffering, even if the result is avoidance and denial.

Candib (1987) spoke about not only the inherent intimacy of patient-doctor relationships but also their reciprocity. She noted that a doctor's sharing his or her own story with a patient can go awry but also can be healing for the doctor, as well as the patient. The question then becomes one of what it means to be involved. Perhaps what the conventional teaching intended to say was: "Don't get involved at the level of your egoistic emotions."

Becoming involved in the right way is crucial to the care of patients but is very difficult in practice. The problem is that none of us are very good at recognizing the many ways in which our egoistic emotions can intrude into our actions (Needleman, 1992). It can take a great moralist like Dostoyevsky or Jane Austen to make us aware of this danger, even when we think we are behaving with the greatest care and compassion. In *The Brothers Karamazov*, Dostoyevsky (1958) described how the young novice monk, Alexey, has tried to give money to a poor man who has been humiliated in public by Alexey's older brother. The man refuses the gift with indignation. Later, Alexey is discussing with Lisa, an invalid girl, how he might get the man to take the money. "Listen Alexey," says Lisa, "don't you think our reasoning . . . shows that we regard him—that unfortunate man—with contempt? I mean that we analyze his soul like this, as though from above? I mean that we're so absolutely certain that he'll accept the money. Don't you think so?" Later in their discussion, Alexey says to her, ". . . your question whether we do not despise that unhappy man by dissecting his soul was the question of a person who has suffered a lot. . . . A person to whom such questions occur is himself capable of suffering" (pp. 252, 254).

In *Emma*, Jane Austen (1981) described how, in a moment of truth, Emma Woodhouse realizes that "with insufferable vanity [she had] believed herself in the secret of everybody's feelings; with unpardonable arrogance proposed to arrange everybody's destiny" (p. 379). Instead of working, as she thought, for the good of her young friend Harriet Smith, she had, in fact, brought evil on her.

Sometimes, at a case conference or videotape review, one has the feeling that the discussion, after starting with the care of the patient, has changed to a dissection from on high of the patient's soul and destiny. The relationship has changed to one in which the physician despises, rather than respects, the patient. Our unrecognized self-absorption can interfere with care in so many ways: our helplessness in the face of suffering, our career commitment to a certain point of view or procedure, our anger when a patient challenges our self-worth, or even when the patient becomes an instrument in our crusade for a worthy cause. Sometimes, our difficulty is a failure to understand that what the patient wants is something very simple: a recognition of his or her suffering or perhaps only our presence at a time of need. For Jane Austen, the key to moral development was always self-knowledge. It is through self-knowledge that we can become involved in the care of patients while avoiding the traps and pitfalls: hence the importance of attending to medicine as a moral education.

Healing

The attributes of the doctor and the characteristics of the relationship are what make the patient-doctor relationship therapeutic. Like many other helping professionals, doctors are experienced as instruments (agents) of healing. This image of the doctor is contained in numerous stories of patients (Stephens, 1993). In particular, Frank (1991) wrote in his book *At the Will of the Body: Reflections on Illness* about his own experience as a patient:

> Medicine has done well with my body and I am grateful. But doing *with* the body is only part of what needs to be done *for* the person. What happens when my body breaks down happens not just to that body but also to my life, which is lived in that body. When the body breaks down, so does the life. Even when medicine can fix the body, that doesn't always put the life back together again. (p. 8)

Healing the body and healing the person are not identical and do not even necessarily go hand in hand. The healing of a patient involves a process of restoring the patient's lost sense of connectedness, indestructibility, and control. The healing process is "no more than allowing, causing or bringing to bear those things or forces for getting better that already exist in the patient" (Cassell, 1991, p. 234).

Physicians, for the most part, see themselves as curers of patients' physical ills. They are less conscious of the need to restore patients to wellness by embracing the mandate to care and to heal. The words *heal, health,* and *whole* all come from the same linguistic root in old English. To heal is to restore a sense of coherence, wholeness, and connectedness after the disruption in a person's life that is caused by a serious illness (Stephens, 1982). After a heart attack at the age of 39 and cancer at 40, Frank wrote about his experience in a health care system that was technically proficient but essentially uncaring. The system seemed to have lost the capacity to heal the patient, as well as treat his body.

Examples of the work of a doctor who recognized the use of the drug "doctor" (Balint, 1957) in a much deeper way than in the previous example are contained in Berger and Mohr's (1967) story of a country doctor, *A Fortunate Man*. Because illness and crises separate people from the ordinariness of the rest of humanity, one requirement of the doctor is to recognize accurately the pain of the patient in order to help restore the patient's lost sense of connectedness and, therefore, to promote healing. This perception not only is difficult to do but also takes courage, a fact that often goes unacknowledged.

> [The country doctor] is acknowledged as a good doctor because he meets the deep but unformulated expectation of the sick for a sense of fraternity. He recognizes them. Sometimes he fails—often because he has missed a critical opportunity and the patient's suppressed resentment becomes too hard to break through—but there is about him the constant will of man trying to recognize. "The door opens," he says, "and sometimes I feel I'm in the valley of death. It's all right when once I'm working. I try to overcome this shyness because for the patient the first contact is extremely important. If he's put off and doesn't feel welcome, it may take a long time to win his confidence back and perhaps never. I try to give him a fully open greeting. All diffidence in my position is a fault. A form of negligence." (pp. 76-77)

Self-Awareness

Whatever use doctors make of themselves and the relationship in caring for patients, it affects them, as well as their patients. Both the use of self and attending to the impact on self require a depth of self-knowledge.

Self-awareness can be a natural outgrowth of reflection on experience and sharing these reflections with colleagues, friends, and family. It can be enhanced further by supervision or consultation, professional and personal development. Epstein et al. (1993) proposed three possible venues for developing self-awareness: (a) Balint groups, which were conceived by Michael and Enid Balint (Balint, 1957) and described by other authors (Frenette & Blondeau, 1989); (b) family of origin groups, stemming from the work of Murray Bowen (1976,

1978), which examine how individuals' families of origin influence their relationships with patients; and (c) personal awareness groups, which evolved from the contributions of Carl Rogers (1961). Other authors endorse the important knowledge and understanding imparted in the classical literature or the insights offered by narratives of illness (Brody, 1992; Kleinman, 1988; McWhinney, 1989c).

Whatever the source, self-awareness and self-knowledge are imperative. As Stein (1985b) observed, "One can truly recognize a patient only if one is willing to recognize oneself in the patient" (p. 31). McWhinney (1989c) had a similar message: "We cannot begin to know others until we know ourselves. We cannot grow and change as physicians until we have removed our defenses and faced up to our shortcomings" (p. 82).

The development of self-awareness requires that doctors know their strengths and weaknesses. What potential blindspots or emotional triggers elicit a negative response to certain patients? As Longhurst (1989) noted, self-awareness means confronting the emotional baggage emanating from our families of origin and conflicts in current relationships. Self-awareness and self-knowledge also have a positive value in that they promote and nurture the qualities of empathy, sensitivity, honesty, and caring in the physician. Because acquiring self-knowledge is often a painful process, this form of knowledge is the most difficult of all to acquire. It is perhaps best seen as a lifelong journey: a process that is never complete.

Transference and Countertransference

All human relationships—and in particular, therapeutic relationships—are influenced by the phenomena of transference and countertransference. Thus any discussion of the patient-doctor relationship that excluded these important psychological processes would be remiss. We do not provide the reader with a detailed examination of transference and countertransference, but rather with a brief description. We think this is essential in order to define the parameters in which many of the dimensions (power, caring, healing, and self-awareness) of the patient-doctor relationship frequently occur.

Transference is a process whereby the patient unconsciously projects onto individuals in his or her current life thoughts, behaviors, and emotional reactions that originate with other significant relationships from childhood onward (Dubovsky, 1981; Hepworth & Larsen, 1990;

Woods & Hollis, 1990). This process can include feelings of love, hate, ambivalence, and dependency. The greater the current attachment, such as a significant patient-doctor relationship, the more likely the transference will occur. Transference, although often perceived as a negative phenomenon, actually helps build the connection between patient and doctor. Frequently, doctors are intimidated by the concept of *transference*, which has its roots in psychoanalytic theory, viewing it as something mysterious and to be avoided. Knowledge of the patient's transference reaction, however, assists the doctor in understanding how the patient experiences his or her world and how past relationships influence current behavior.

Transference can occur during any stage of the patient-doctor relationship and can be activated by any number of events. For example, when the capabilities of seriously ill patients are impaired or when patients are overwhelmed by the ramifications implied by a specific diagnosis, they may respond to their doctor in an uncharacteristic manner. They may return to a position of dependency and neediness, which is more a reflection of unresolved past relationships than of their current relationship with the physician. Patients may seek, during this time of crisis, the care and comfort that was absent in their past. Conversely, they may respond by becoming distant and aloof, indicating the return to a stoical stance adopted in their early years, when they were forced to assume a position of pseudoindependence and self-sufficiency. A doctor's inadvertent failure to respond to a patient's need or request may evoke unwarranted anger or hostility. It is imperative to understand the genesis of the patient's response, which may originate from years of feeling misunderstood and uncared for. Understanding the patient's transference reactions enhances the doctor's capacity for caring and can provide an emotional corrective experience. It also can circumvent abuses of power in the patient-doctor relationship when patients are vulnerable and in need of caring and compassion.

Stein (1985a) noted "how rarely the issue of physician countertransference was addressed in medical school, residency training, or continuing education" (p. xii). He believes that "most of the problems in clinician-patient relationships did not have to do with technical or procedural issues in patient management but with those unconscious agendas which physicians and patients brought to the encounter" (p. xii). Like transference, countertransference is an unconscious process that occurs when the doctor responds to patients in a manner similar to significant past relationships (Dubovsky, 1981; Hepworth

& Larsen, 1990; Woods & Hollis, 1990). Doctors need to be alert to what triggers certain reactions (unresolved personal issues, stress, or value conflicts). It is here that self-awareness, coupled with the ability for self-observation during the consultation, is paramount.

Some of the commonly agreed on signs of countertransference are touched on in our description of the first three components of patient-centered practice—for example, not listening attentively, interpreting too soon, misjudging the patient's level of feeling, becoming too active in giving advice, becoming overly identified with the patient's problem, gaining vicarious pleasure in the patient's story, engaging in power struggles with the patient, running late, running overtime, and covering the same material with the patient over and over (Dubovsky, 1981; Hepworth & Larsen, 1990).

The origins and significance of doctors' countertransference are as varied and complex as their patients. As noted earlier in this chapter, we all struggle with unresolved issues from our past. For example, the doctor who finds himself repeatedly giving advice to depressed female patients may be attempting to rescue the patients from their sorrow in a way similar to how he responded to his own mother's chronic angst. The constant inability to listen to a patient's painful story of failed relationships may relate to parallel experiences in the doctor's own life. The demanding and obstinate behaviors of a patient, in turn, activate behaviors by the physician, such as running late, avoidance, or engaging in power struggles, all responses that may have been characteristic of the doctor's relationship with a domineering father.

Stein (1985a) observed that the most common subjects of medical countertransference are "intensely personal ones that correspond to the culturally most vexatious emotional issues as well: aggression, death, loss, grief, separation, sexuality, intimacy, control, autonomy, dependency, self-reliance, time, and integrity of the self (for example, self/other boundaries)" (p. 28).

The primary tool for effectively using transference and countertransference to aid and deepen the patient-physician relationship is physician self-awareness. Such self-knowledge is a requirement for the doctor's accurate recognition of both transference and countertransference. Self-evaluation and working with others may help doctors gain valuable insights that ultimately will strengthen relationships with patients and also increase their own comfort and satisfaction with the practice of medicine.

CONTROL AND REASSURANCE

Case Illustrating Component 5: Enhancing the Relationship

Moira Stewart

Judith Belle Brown

W. Wayne Weston

Mrs. P. was an elderly woman who had arthritis, irritable bowel syndrome, and a cancer of the breast 6 years ago. The doctor, in his late 30s, had been Mrs. P.'s family physician for the past 2 years.

Patient: Good morning, Doctor. Now, the first thing I want to deal with is this funny pain in my back. *(Whenever I get a pain, I worry about the cancer coming back. I feel silly to say it out loud.)*

The physician clarified the description of the pain and examined Mrs. P.

Doctor: Well, Mrs. P., the pain seems to me to be typical muscular pain, probably from the lawn bowling you started last week. I'm satisfied that this is nothing other then muscle pain and not anything like a recurrence of the cancer, but if you want, we can arrange an X-ray. *(I know I cannot be 100% sure, but I also think that Mrs. P. needs me to be definite in my reassurance.)*

Patient: Oh, if you're satisfied, then I am too. *(Thank heaven he isn't like the doctor I had who always left me feeling unsure.)* If you're finished, then, let's go to the next item on my list.

Doctor: OK. Go ahead. *(Hmmmm. One minute she needs me to be in charge and be certain, and in the next minute she wants to take charge.)*

This insightful patient and doctor found a way to accommodate her seemingly contradictory needs. On the one hand, her advanced age and physical problems left her insecure enough to require explicit reassurance. The doctor provided the reassurance after appropriate questioning and physical examination and by exploring the nature of her pain. On the other hand, she needed to maintain control over some aspects of her life; this manifested itself in her controlling the choice and the order of topics during the encounter with her family doctor. Although this physician thoughtfully interpreted her behavior, other professionals might have been offended by her somewhat bossy manner and might have failed to see it as a coping mechanism.

Studies have shown that elderly patients have different expectations of their doctor than younger adult patients; they wanted more information about their condition, but they did not want to share the decision making with the doctor (Beisecker & Beisecker, 1990; Ende, Kazis, Ash, & Moskowitz, 1989). It may not be the case that physicians communicate in the same way with all patients regardless of their age and expectations. Early work of Byrne and Long (1976) found that doctors' styles of communicating were somewhat rigid. More recent work has indicated that although some physicians are consistent in their communication, others show a variety of approaches, perhaps depending on the needs of the individual patient (Stewart et al., 1989). Ende et al. (1989) recommended that "for the clinician it is perhaps more important to recognize and accommodate the preferences of individual patients, which can vary considerably from one patient to the next" (p. 27) and, one could add, for a given patient from one moment to the next.

Subtle cues from patients may provide guides to the doctor regarding the degree of control or the degree of support they need. Beisecker and Beisecker (1990) observed that patients, in reciprocal manner, take cues about appropriate role behavior from their doctors. Other situational variables, such as diagnosis, reason for the visit, and time constraints, may have influenced the cues.

The case presented above illustrates how, in one visit, the patient's preference for control oscillated from one moment to the next. One could imagine that this seeming contradiction may have had the potential of leaving a doctor feeling confused, frustrated, and resentful of the patient.

Mrs. P. explicitly let her doctor know that she needed to deal with her "list" in her order. In the following visit, the patient stated, "Doctor, the best thing you did at my last visit was let me go through my whole list." Not all patients are so insightful as to know and express their needs so clearly. Indeed, Mrs. P. did not make her need for reassurance so explicit. She recognized it but was too embarrassed to reveal it. For this need, the doctor relied on being completely open and attentive to his patient to facilitate recognition of subtle verbal and nonverbal cues. The doctor recognized the importance of split-second alternating back and forth in his role as take-charge clinician and acquiescent supporter of her initiatives in order to meet Mrs. P.'s needs and to reassure her. Finally, this case illustrates a physician who used his knowledge of himself and the patient to engage in an evolving and healing relationship.

NOTE: This case description first appeared in the April 1993 issue of the *Ontario Medical Review* and is reprinted with the permission of the Ontario Medical Association.

8

The Sixth Component

Being Realistic

JUDITH BELLE BROWN

CAROL L. McWILLIAM

W. WAYNE WESTON

Patient problems are increasingly more complex and multifaceted, time is scarce, resources are at a premium, doctors' physical and emotional energies are constantly taxed, and the increasing demands of bureaucracy are often overwhelming. In this chapter, we examine the issue of being realistic in terms of what a single practitioner can reasonably expect to achieve in providing patient-centered care, given normal human limitations. We examine issues of time, accessing resources, team building, and the importance of wise stewardship.

Time and Timing

We contend that visits in which an understanding of disease and illness is gained, an understanding of the whole person is achieved, and the patient and the doctor find common ground are not necessarily lengthy visits. Indeed, research has shown that visits in which the patients are active participants in telling about their illness and in asking questions are almost identical in length to other visits—30 minutes in U.S. primary care internal medicine offices (Greenfield et al., 1988) and 9 minutes in Canadian family practices (Stewart et al., 1989).

Furthermore, such visits are likely to be the best use of resources over the long term, potentially saving the patient from having to return to receive a more accurate recognition of the problems and leading to fewer unnecessary tests and referrals because the problems have been more appropriately prioritized.

We do not suggest that all areas of patient concern be explored in every visit. In fact, one of the strong points of medical care is the possibility of using several visits, over time, to explore complex or deeply personal issues. Often, after a close and trusting relationship has developed, doctor and patient can get to the heart of a matter very quickly. Thus time and timing are two key factors.

Although it is not realistic to deal with all of the problems of every patient in each visit, doctors must be able to recognize when a patient requires more time, even if it means disrupting their office schedules. When a patient presents with multiple symptoms and concerns, the physician must learn how to establish which are the most pressing issues at that time. This assessment requires that the doctor learn how to prioritize the patient's problems, guided by the patient's expressed concerns and the potential seriousness of the problems. When the patient's or another's safety may be at risk, the doctor may need to take a more assertive role in this process. For example, child abuse, suicidal ideation, woman abuse, and life-threatening medical situations, such as ketoacidosis or asthma, require urgent attention.

It is important for the physician to address the patient's problem in the most effective and efficient manner and to pave the way for the patient to return to the office to explore the remaining concerns. In adopting this prioritizing approach, the doctor must learn how to create quickly an atmosphere in which patients feel heard and understand that the doctor sees their problems as important and worthy of further exploration. If patients leave the office feeling frustrated, they may not pursue their remaining concerns during subsequent visits. Alternatively, a patient's "symptoms" may intensify and be presented through multiple visits in an attempt to "prompt" the doctor about unresolved concerns. In either scenario, the interactions that transpire will be unsatisfactory and unfulfilling for both patient and doctor.

Perhaps most frustrating for physicians is the "doorknob" comment by patients—that singular comment as the patient leaves the visit, hand on the office doorknob, that alerts the doctor to a complex web of pain, either physical, emotional, or social. Again, the doctor needs to acknowledge the patient's concern. Depending on time and availability, the problem may be addressed at that moment, or arrangements should be secured for further follow-up about the problem. If the doctor fails to elicit the patient's underlying concerns, the potential outcome may be an unnecessary use of resources at subsequent visits. The result may be increased cost to an already overburdened health care system. In search of an answer perceived to fit the problem, the patient may demand further visits, additional investigations, and often unwarranted procedures, leaving both patient and doctor dissatisfied.

Essential skills needed by the doctor are flexibility and a readiness to express both concern and a willingness to work with the patient in the future. Doctors need to work with patients to establish mutual agreement. This applies to both defining the problem and deciding the most realistic treatment or management plan to avoid misuse of resources. The following case illustrates some of these key points.

CASE EXAMPLE

Mr. O., 75 years old, was admitted to the hospital with pneumonia, a complication of long-standing chronic obstructive pulmonary disease. His physical symptoms had necessitated nebulized ventolin therapy by mask. Just prior to discharge from the hospital, the specialist and his team had decided to switch Mr. O.'s treatment to a self-administered inhaler, which was more practical for use at home. Mr. O., distressed by this new treatment approach, tried unsuccessfully to make his physicians understand his concerns. "I just can't get this stuff in. I can't inhale!" he exclaimed. Even after the use of a spacer was carefully explained, he still felt overwhelmed. As the time to return home approached, he became increasingly anxious, expressing fear that he would not be able to breathe well enough to resume the daily chores he undertook as part of caring for his frail wife.

At home, Mr. O. continued to suffer from his respiratory symptoms. Ever conscious of his family responsibilities, Mr. O. struggled unsuccessfully to follow medical instructions to regain weight. Eating had become a "tremendous chore" because of his respiratory problems. Unable to resume his customary homemaking duties, Mr. O. became progressively demoralized. He felt totally misunderstood by his physician, who explained: "The puffers haven't been shown to be any less effective. The only difference is psychological." Mr. O. disagreed, saying, "I know you can't tell the doctors how to treat you, but I don't think it is psychological. The problems I have with trying to clear phlegm from my throat before I can eat my meal is certainly not psychological! . . . I will tell you one thing for sure. It rules out all of the relatively simple things that you used to be able to do." Mr. O.'s lack of confidence in his ability to use the hand-held nebulizer was aggravated by his feeling that the doctor did not understand his problem. He became more anxious, and his general condition deteriorated.

As a consequence of the doctor's failure to grasp the implications of his prescribed treatment plan, precious time and resources were consumed. Additional professional home care services were required, and Mr. O. eventually had to be rehospitalized. Apparent efficiency did not translate into effective patient-centered care.

Timing also speaks to the issue of the patient's readiness to share certain concerns or experiences with the doctor. Reluctance to present concerns may arise for a variety of reasons. In such circumstances, the doctor's knowledge of the whole person can be of vital importance in understanding patients. For example, patients may be reluctant to disclose family problems because disclosure runs counter to family norms and values—"These problems are our business, and no one else needs to know about them!" Some patients may feel an intense loyalty to family members and, as a result, believe that seeking help is an act of betrayal that could lead to rejection or isolation from the family. But keeping the family secrets denies them what they need most—help and understanding.

Patients are often reticent to share their concerns or problems for fear of reprisal or abandonment by the doctor. They may experience their inability to resolve their problems independently as a failure or a loss of face. As a result, patients often feel shame, embarrassment, or anxiety when seeking help. Especially in the primary care setting, it may take them several visits with the doctor, frequently marked by undifferentiated physical complaints, before they can reveal the actual source of their concern. When they finally do share their understanding of the problem with their doctor, it may be on an occasion when the doctor is pressed for time or emotionally worn by the demands of the practice. Again, it is important for the doctor to acknowledge the patient's concerns and to provide an environment that lends itself to further exploration of the problem. It may not be realistic or even wise to delve extensively into the problem at this time. When a doctor is exhausted from long, sleepless nights on call, it is often wise to acknowledge the fatigue, both to him- or herself and to the patients, and to ask whether the patients would be willing to return when the doctor is rested and better able to help. It is essential that patients feel understood and know the doctor is prepared to work with them on their problems during future visits. This knowledge will be supported and enhanced by the strength of the patient-doctor relationship.

Accessing Resources and Team Building

Expecting doctors to be knowledgeable about every available resource in their community for each specific group they serve is simply not realistic. For example, doctors may not be knowledgeable about all available support groups for all disease entities and all cultural groups. Nevertheless, they must be prepared to learn about the context in which their patients live and how to access the appropriate resources. Thus the issue is not one of knowing the specific resources, but of knowing the key personnel who can locate, motivate, and promote change. It is reasonable to expect that doctors know whom they can access to locate needed resources—for example, who can advocate for their patient about housing, who can recommend an appropriate support group, who can facilitate a referral to a local rehabilitation program, and who can mediate between the bureaucracy of the welfare system and the patient. Exercising such knowledge may require that the doctor orchestrate a "team" and adopt a position of shared responsibility and power.

Orchestrating a multidisciplinary team is often a difficult task for doctors, who have assumed a "lone ranger" approach to practice (Lee, 1980; Poulton & West, 1993). As McWhinney (1989c) noted, "No one profession can meet all of patients' needs, hence the need to work together in teams. There are strengths, but also pitfalls, in teamwork. There are also misconceptions about what teamwork is" (p. 343).

The concept of shared power or responsibility may seem, at best, foreign and, at worst, formidable (Huffman, 1993). But teams can assist doctors in not becoming overextended and in limiting responsibilities to what realistically can be achieved. The challenge for many doctors may come with the initial questions: How do you formulate such a team? How do you "share" responsibility for patient care?

A framework for sharing responsibilities among multiple care-givers affords three approaches to successful team building: co-ordination, cooperation, and collaboration. With the *coordination* approach, the doctor assumes a "linchpin" position, serving as the coordinator of services (Huffman, 1993). This includes bringing together the necessary services or personnel to meet patient needs. The doctor draws on the expertise of various health care professionals (e.g., nurses, social workers, psychologists, and clergy) and delegates tasks appropriate to each discipline. This approach serves as a useful strategy when health care professionals seek to avoid unnecessary competition or duplication in their care of patients.

Coordination promotes the achievement of multiple goals and tasks in health care delivery by multiple participants (Baggs & Schmitt, 1988). However, the coordination approach has several disadvantages. This manner of care compartmentalizes health care delivery, assigning each group specific tasks or responsibilities. The drawback for the busy practitioner may be the demands of coordinating such an effort. In the absence of full knowledge of the involvement of other health and social service agencies, duplication of services or gaps in service may result. From the patient's perspective, the consequences may be fragmented care and confusion about accessing and using the appropriate resources.

The *cooperation* approach brings together a large group of professionals for an exchange of ideas and information (Germain, 1984). In many ways, it is similar to the traditional case conference in which several health care professionals gather at a designated time to discuss specific patient problems or management issues. Each participant works independently but in concert with other members to address particular patient needs. Two major difficulties arise with the cooperative strategy. First, the approach tends to be case specific. Second, the approach does not ensure integrated team functioning. Much time and effort may be consumed in negotiating professional roles and extent of involvement (Lowe & Herranen, 1978). Patients can experience fragmented care and confusion about service delivery as a result.

In contrast to the preceding options, the *collaboration* approach tends to be more flexible and crosses disciplinary boundaries. It capitalizes on the talents and expertise of all professionals involved. This approach requires a more equitable distribution of responsibility and power. It means that all professionals involved in the patient's care assume an equal degree of responsibility and accountability for the services being provided. Professional activities may cross traditional roles and functions, but ultimately they lead to increased comprehensive patient care (Schlesinger, 1985). The collaborative approach entails greater blurring of team members' roles with involvement premised on who can best meet the patient's needs at that moment. This may be determined by specific care needs or influenced by the quality of the relationship between the patient and a particular member of the team. Critical to the collaborative approach is the active involvement of patients in all phases of planning and implementing their care; they are viewed as equal participants on the health care team. An environment of working together with a common cause—patient well-being—is the primary goal.

In the previous chapter, on enhancing the patient-doctor relationship, we highlighted the importance of practitioners developing self-awareness. Being aware of one's own strengths and weaknesses guides the doctor in seeking help and support with problems that are baffling or difficult. Requesting assistance or consultation with other professionals should not be viewed as a deficit in knowledge or ability, but as an opportunity for further learning and growth. This approach also can provide the doctor with new information and offer a different perspective on the problem. Although a team approach initially may seem time-consuming and not particularly cost effective, seeking guidance can reduce the doctor's frustration, confusion, and emotional depletion. Ultimately, both physician renewal and improved patient care often result.

Wise Stewardship

Doctors currently are challenged by issues of cost containment and increasing bureaucratic demands, all of which infringe on patient-centered practice (Miller, 1993). Health care systems, like all bureaucracies, are notorious for their red tape, one-way flow of information, centralized control, and fragmented services. Although efficiency, the ultimate goal of bureaucratic structure, often appears greatest in the larger, more bureaucratic health care organization (Hummel, 1987), effective care delivery is often undermined, especially in the larger, more complex urban teaching hospital setting (McWilliam & Sangster, 1994; McWilliam & Wong, 1994). People, politics, location, and happenstance can and do influence decisions and priorities, necessitating the doctor's attention to stewardship and patient advocacy (Brody, 1992). All of these characteristics necessitate that the doctor spend more time in communication and coordination of care (McWilliam & Sangster, 1994).

Above all, the bureaucratic health care context has, over the years, influenced patient-doctor relationships (Siegler, 1985). Paternalistic approaches of the past have been replaced in recent years by a focus on autonomy. Recent pressures for economical practice, however, have threatened the patient-doctor relationship. The doctor is now increasingly pulled by the system to consider the needs of hospitals and other health care agencies, of health care system employees, and of society in general, along with considering the patient's needs. Some suggest that "the wishes of both patients and physicians are already or soon will be subservient to the wishes of government bureaucrats, administrators of Health Maintenance Organizations, insurance company executives or corporate vice-presidents of proprietary multi-hospital chains" (Siegler, 1985, p. 715). Coping with the growing demands of bureaucracy and its threat to patient-centered care requires constant conscious attention to the realities of the evolving health care system. Doctors must ensure that patient-centeredness and the patient-physician relationship do not suffer in the process of making trade-offs.

There are limitations to the fiduciary role assigned to physicians, yet they need to practice wise stewardship of the limited community resources. Meeting the needs of all constituencies demands creating a balance between the needs of the individual patient and the needs of the community. Doctors cannot avoid the conflict of interest inherent in resource management. Therefore, part of being realistic is constantly making a conscious choice in determining value trade-offs between patients' needs and wants and the resources available. It is a taxing part of professional judgment but should not occur by default.

Conclusion

Being realistic about patient-centered care necessitates mastery of several elements of the art of medical practice. Learning the best timing and time allotment for problems is essential. Accessing resources and effective team building also contribute to practicing realistically. Awareness of one's own abilities and priorities both as a practitioner and as a person is critical to orchestrating a team approach. Currently, issues of cost containment and increasing demands of bureaucracy create the need for wise stewardship of the health care system's resources.

We do not pretend to have all the answers. This would be impossible, given the rapid and radical changes continuously occurring in the health care system. Flexibility and a willingness to explore the most appropriate options available for practice are a never-ending necessity. The ideas we present are relevant to today but will need to be adapted to the changing environment and all of the societal, economic, cultural, and health issues that confront us in the future.

"SHOW ME THE WAY TO GO HOME"

Case Illustrating Component 6:
Being Realistic

Carol L. McWilliam

Judith Belle Brown

John Yaphe

They keep changing it around! . . . You don't know whether you're coming or going! I said to Dr. P., "I don't give a damn!" The last time I was here, they kept me here 4 months!

Mr. S., a 77-year-old bachelor with chronic obstructive pulmonary disease, was referred by his family physician to a surgeon and subsequently was admitted to a general hospital for a simple mastectomy to remove a small lump on the breast. Assessment for surgery revealed severe uncontrolled diabetes mellitus. Thus a medical internist, a surgeon, and a family physician attended Mr. S. during his hospitalization.

Surgery and medical care progressed without complication, and Mr. S.'s family physician advised that he had recuperated sufficiently for discharge. As the designated attending physician, he wrote the discharge order, specifying diabetic classes, home care referral, and an office appointment in 3 weeks. Delighted at the prospect of returning home to the company of old friends eager to plan their annual spring fishing expedition, Mr. S. made arrangements for his sister to pick him up at the hospital.

111

Unfortunately, however, both Mr. S. and his family physician had misunderstood arrangements for diabetic classes. Both thought these could be pursued on an outpatient basis. Such was not the case. The nurse-in-charge corrected this misunderstanding, confirming a stay of an additional week in the hospital to complete diabetic classes. Mr. S. reluctantly but good-humoredly accepted this delay.

In the middle of the week of diabetic instruction, Mr. S.'s surgeon visited, commented positively on Mr. S.'s progress, and observed that he certainly was now fit for discharge. With an enthusiastic eye on the spring day outside and with a head filled with thoughts of fine fishing, Mr. S. heard a comment that fulfilled his wishful thinking. Thus, the next day, when his attending family physician confirmed that he had written an order for discharge on the following day, Mr. S. quickly moved once again to make arrangements for his sister to retrieve him from the hospital. As he packed his belongings in anticipation of discharge on the following day, Mr. S. told his hospital roommate animated stories of annual fishing trips with his buddies for the past 22 years.

The following day, however, was a Friday. That morning, Mr. S.'s internist made rounds and stopped in to see Mr. S., who related his excitement about discharge, conveying plans that did not emphasize much concern about his diabetic regimen. The internist, familiar with Mr. S. from having provided many years of care for his COPD, became understandably alarmed. He feared discharge of Mr. S. on a Friday, without adequate weekend coverage by home care professionals who could monitor his diabetic regimen and respond to any related care needs. The internist took great pains to explain this concern to Mr. S. and then proceeded to cancel the discharge order.

Although he accepted the physician's decision, Mr. S. was extremely disappointed. Planning the annual fishing trip was a ritual in many ways as exciting as the trip itself. And now, for the first time in 22 years, he would not be with his three friends for this weekend's planning session. What was perhaps worse, in his mind, was that although he was the youngest of this foursome, he was the first to miss this event. Thus, when the home care case manager visited him that morning, Mr. S. was despondent. In his estimation, she had let him down because it was she who arranged postdischarge professional services in the home. Mr. S. vividly recounted the details of this whole discharge experience with a tone of resigned exasperation and some bitterness.

This story highlights the challenges of achieving patient-centered care. Excellent communication between each individual professional and the patient does not ensure excellent care, despite the expertise and concern of each professional caregiver. Communication is multidimensional, and patient-centered care in hospitals always involves many professionals. In the absence of deliberate effort to coordinate care by several professionals, the patient often receives mixed or conflicting messages. Perceived care then can amount to less than the sum total of the care provided by individual practitioners.

To achieve patient-centered care in our complex health care system, a coordinated multidisciplinary approach is necessary (O'Hare & Terry, 1988). Someone must take responsibility for understanding each patient's unique situation and for tailoring the interventions of all involved to meet the patient's unique needs (Pfeiffer, 1985). Care of the elderly often presents particular challenges. This approach requires an ongoing team effort, with regular, open communication and shared decision making about care plans. Family physicians frequently coordinate services for their patients when several physicians are involved in their care (O'Hare & Terry, 1988). Most important, patients themselves need to be involved in a meaningful way if deliberations are to achieve and communicate coordinated care (Balint, 1964).

Fortunately, good communication among involved professionals created a happy ending for this story. The home care case manager immediately conferred with Mr. S.'s internist and family physician. Together, the three decided that weekend coverage with professional home care services was appropriate, and discharge therefore was reordered for that day. Through coordination of their individual efforts to provide quality care to the patient, these professionals were able to achieve effective patient-centered care.

NOTE: This case description first appeared in the April 1992 issue of the *Ontario Medical Review* and is reprinted with the permission of the Ontario Medical Association.

PART TWO

Learning and Teaching

9

Teaching the Patient-Centered Method

The Human Dimensions of Medical Education

W. WAYNE WESTON

JUDITH BELLE BROWN

M any of us have seen the famous painting by Luke Fildes of the physician at the bedside of a seriously ill child with her parents standing, worrying, in the dark shadows in the background. This mythological image depicts the country doctor waging war against disease single-handedly, with no other tools except those that can be carried in the doctor's bag. It is a popular image of caring and compassion that appeals to our longing for an all-powerful healer.

But there is another way to see this picture—through the eyes of a young physician. What does he or she see?—a doctor, with no laboratory or X-ray machine to confirm the diagnosis, with no drug to cure the problem, with no way to alter the natural course of the disease, and with no one to refer the patient to. It is a terrifying prospect for many graduates who carefully avoid moving to small communities where they fear they might face situations like this.

AUTHORS' NOTE: The authors thank Oxford University Press for permission to quote from E. J. Cassell (1991), *The nature of suffering and the goals of medicine*.

This fear is ironic because, even in large medical centers, physicians frequently confront the limits of medical science. Ingelfinger (1980) stated that 90% of the time, when a patient consults a doctor, either the patient's condition is self-limited or no treatment can alter the natural history of the disease. Much of the time, the most important thing that doctors have to offer their patients is themselves—their time, their interest, and their understanding.

In a study of 272 patients presenting to their family doctors with headaches in London, Canada, the Headache Study Group (1986) looked for what would predict a favorable outcome 1 year later. Investigation, treatment, and referral were all unrelated. The best outcomes were in patients who thought they had been given sufficient opportunity to tell the doctor all they wanted to say about their headaches on the initial visit. Another predictor of good outcome was the doctor's statement that he or she liked the patient.

Glasser and Pelto (1980) presented the dilemma for medical educators who recognize that physician effectiveness often relates to their personal qualities: "It is rather tragic: modern physicians are a type of shaman without the proper upbringing. It is rather like being Jewish as a third generation American and not knowing how to read or sing Hebrew. It is as though we physicians do not know the prayers and chants" (p. 24). How can physicians learn these "prayers and chants"? What does educational theory offer to guide educators responsible for the development of the modern "shamans"? The patient-centered method describes a different way of doctoring; consequently, education about the method requires a different way of teaching. In this chapter, we describe a framework that addresses this challenge—a framework that builds on the distinction between traditional conceptions of teaching and several ways of understanding the human experience of learning a profession.

Two Metaphors Used in Teaching

Teaching is too complex to be embraced by a single model. Medical education, like medicine itself, embraces opposing theories. Tiberius (1986) outlined two common metaphors used to describe teaching:

1. The *transmission metaphor* dominates all levels of education. In this metaphor, teaching is telling, and learning is listening. The em-

phasis is on the efficient flow of information *down the pipeline* to the students. Examples of this metaphor in common speech are:

It is hard to *get* that idea *across* to him.

Your reasons come *through* to us.

Delivery of material.

2. The *metaphor of dialogue or conversation* has roots in the Socratic method and the humanist tradition. In this metaphor, students and teachers are "inquirers, helping one another in the shared pursuit of truth. . . . They are engaged in a common enterprise in which the responsibility for acquiring knowledge is a joint one" (Hendley, 1978, p. 144). "Education . . . is not a bunch of tricks or even a bundle of knowledge. Education is something we neither 'give' nor 'do' to our students. Rather, *it is a way we stand in relation to them*" (Daloz, 1986, p. xv).

The dialogue metaphor recognizes that becoming a physician is more than simply learning a set of knowledge, skills, and attitudes; medical training not only teaches a body of knowledge but also changes the person. In this sense, medical education is as much about the acquisition of values and character development as it is about learning a discipline. Unfortunately, although these issues have been acknowledged for generations, medical education is often inimical to healthy personal development.

The following vignette illustrates the challenges inherent in the application of the dialogue metaphor. One of us (Weston), many years ago, learned the hard way about the importance of personal factors in teaching and learning.

One of my postgraduate students had a very different idea of what he wanted to learn from what I wanted to teach. He worried about being able to deal effectively with emergencies, but I wanted him to learn more about interviewing and the patient-doctor relationship. We often debated about the proper role of family doctors, and each of us stubbornly clung to our own point of view. While he was away doing hospital rotations, he sent me a book to read, a book that he said had meant a great deal to him in his adolescence. He thought it might help me understand him better. I started to read it but found it so at variance with my own worldview that I could not finish it. Later, he urged me to see the movie *Chariots of Fire*. He explained that he strongly identified with the main character in the film at the point when the Prince of Wales was called in to persuade him to "bend" his strong Christian principles by running a race on a Sunday. I thought he must be exaggerating and had trouble equating his struggles with the moral issues in the story. He then shared with me how he grappled to assert his identity and his conflict with his authoritarian father. Despite our attempts to understand each other, we continued to disagree about what he should learn. He eventually graduated and set up a successful rural practice. A few years later, I met him at a dinner party; we immediately struck up a conversation, talking for more than an hour about his experiences since graduation. He told me that I had been right; he handled emergencies without trouble but still experienced difficulty helping patients with emotional problems. On his own, he gradually was learning how to help them. It was an emotional and very special meeting for both of us. We learned a lot from each other about our stubbornness and our need to be in charge. Through our struggles with each other, we were challenged to reexamine the roles of the physician and the goals of postgraduate education. But, more important, our encounters showed us a different way for teacher and learner to relate to one another; we had to move beyond an authoritarian model that provoked resistance to a model of dialogue that respected the contributions of each person. This change, this different way of relating, illustrates a learner-centered approach that is a conceptual parallel with the patient-centered method. Both approaches seek a partnership between the protagonists—patient and doctor or student and teacher—characterized by mutual respect that leads to finding common ground.

Understanding the
Human Dimensions of Learning

In becoming physicians, students pass through three phases:

1. *Gaining technical competence in dealing with disease.* This is the principal preoccupation of the 4 years of medical school. Students are immersed in the biological sciences and quickly learn the value system of the medical establishment: The primary task of medicine is the recognition and treatment of disease. Everything else—commu-

nication, psychological, social, and environmental factors—become peripheral. One result of this arrangement is the deterioration of students' ability to communicate effectively with patients as they progress through medical school (Barbee & Feldman, 1970; Cohen, 1985; Helfer, 1970; Preven, Kachur, Kupfer, & Waters, 1986).

2. *Developing a professional identity.* This phase usually is begun during clinical clerkship and completed during residency training. It is only when students work as part of the clinical team and have responsibility for patient care that they begin to feel like doctors. The metamorphosis is dramatic; students usually become comfortable with their strengths and limitations, develop a clearer sense of their professional roles, and refine their ability to appraise critically their own performance (Brent, 1981).

3. *Learning to heal.* During this phase, physicians learn to be instruments of healing, accepting with humility and wisdom the power to heal bestowed on them by their patients. This phase takes at least 5 to 10 years and is not accomplished by all physicians. Cassell (1991) challenged us to address the responsibility of medicine to heal:

It has been one of the most basic errors of the modern era in medicine to believe that patients cured of their diseases—cancer removed, coronary arteries opened, infection resolved, walking again, talking again, or back home again—are also healed; are whole again. Through the relationship it is possible, given the awareness of the necessity, the acceptance of the moral responsibility, the understanding of the problem and mastery of the skills, to heal the sick; to make whole the cured, to bring the chronically ill back within the fold, to relieve suffering, and to lift the burdens of illness. (p. 69)

It is important to note that learning to be a healer continues after formal education is completed. The seeds are planted during the training period but only grow and develop as physicians experience the power of the healing relationship in practice. When teachers introduce the concept of healing, they need to be cautious about the expectations they place on their students. These young physicians often find the tasks of diagnosing and treating the biological dimensions of their patients' problems challenging enough; pushing them to become therapeutic instruments of healing may leave them overwhelmed. They need frequent encouragement, support, effective role modeling, and opportunities to discuss their feelings and internal struggles to adopt the healer's mantle.

To help their students negotiate these three phases of development, teachers need a conceptual framework that will guide their understanding of the human dimensions of medical education. A confluence of writings from several directions provides us with valuable insights:

1. *Learning as a transformational journey.* A remarkable number of students have described their personal experiences and struggles in medical school, including a former professor of medicine (Eichna, 1980), an educational psychologist (Eisner, 1985), an anthropologist (Konner, 1987), and others (Klass, 1987, 1992; Klitzman, 1989; LeBaron, 1981; Little & Midtling, 1989; Reilly, 1987).

2. *Developmental theory.* The recent works of psychologists in adult development (Brookfield, 1986; Chickering, 1981; Knowles, 1984, 1986, 1989; Merriam & Caffarella, 1991) provide valuable frameworks for understanding the professional development of physicians.

3. *Mentoring.* Levinson (1978), Daloz (1986), and others (e.g., Baskett & Marsick, 1992) have described the teacher-learner relationship as a mentoring relationship. This concept leads to a number of practical suggestions for improving one-to-one teaching.

4. *The nature of clinical problems.* Schon (1983, 1987) introduced a new educational paradigm rooted in a practical analysis of the professional's role. He argued that learning to think like a practitioner requires a new approach to teaching and curriculum design that addresses the "messiness" of daily professional practice.

In the remainder of the chapter, we elaborate on each of these four areas.

LEARNING AS A TRANSFORMATIONAL JOURNEY

One of the central tasks in our development is to find the meaning of our lives. One way to do this is by telling stories. "The narrative structure is one of the most basic ways we make sense of our experience" (Daloz, 1986, p. 22). Common to hundreds of myths and legends across numerous cultures and times is the tale of the heroic quest: "The hero ventures forth from the world of common day into a region of supernatural wonder: fabulous forces are there encountered and a decisive victory is won: the hero comes back from this mysterious adventure with the power to bestow boons on his fellow-man" (Campbell in Daloz, 1986, p. 25).

Through the "heroic quest" of medical school, the student conquers many "fabulous forces" and becomes a physician: He or she is transformed. Perri Klass (1987) described her experience at Harvard Medical School in these terms:

> The general pressure of medical school is to push yourself ahead into professionalism, to start feeling at home in the hospital, in the operating room, to make medical jargon your native tongue; it's all part of becoming efficient, knowledgeable, competent. You want to leave behind that green, terrified medical student who stood awkwardly on the edge of the action, terrified of revealing limitless ignorance, terrified of killing a patient. You want to identify with the people ahead of you, the ones who know what they are doing. . . . One of the sad effects of my clinical training was that I think I generally became a more impatient, unpleasant person. Time was precious, sleep was often insufficient, and in the interest of my evaluations, I had to treat all kinds of turkeys with profound respect. (p. 18)

Another medical student, Melvin Konner, had been a professor of anthropology prior to his attending medical school. He described his experiences as follows:

> And of course, last but hardly least, I now tend to see people as patients. I noticed this especially with women. It is often asked whether male medical students become desexualized by all those women disrobing, all those breast examinations, all those manual invasions of the most intimate cavities. I found that to be a rather trivial effect. What I found more impressive was the general tendency to see women as patients. This clinical detachment comes not from gynaecology but from all the experiences of medicine. I described a time during my medical station when, on a bus, I noticed the veins on a woman's hand—how easily they could be punctured for the insertion of a line—before noticing that she happened to be beautiful. (Konner, 1987, p. 366)

Both examples illustrate how the journey through medical school may desensitize students to human suffering; they become more impatient and detached. The experience of postgraduate training may be even more brutalizing, leaving young physicians feeling abused. Evidence suggests that students who feel abused by their teachers are more likely to abuse their patients (Baldwin, Daugherty, & Eckenfels, 1991; Silver & Glicken, 1990). Such an environment is inimical to learning to be patient-centered.

DEVELOPMENTAL THEORY

Developmental theory provides a way of understanding learning, not simply as the accumulation of knowledge but also as a transformational experience. Klass (1987) and Konner (1987) described their own experiences of being changed, of no longer being able to see the world "through preclinical eyes."

Perry (1970, 1981) provided a theory of intellectual and ethical development in adult students that is helpful for making sense of these changes in thinking and perceiving. According to Perry, students progress from thinking that is simplistic and "black and white" to where they recognize and can accept different points of view. In the first stage, students view knowledge as dualistic: There is one right answer, determined by the authorities. Next, students recognize different perspectives to issues but are unable to evaluate them; then students develop an ability to critically compare different viewpoints and make their own judgments. Finally, a stage of commitment is attained in which the learners are willing to act according to their values and beliefs even when plausible alternatives are recognized. Students recognize that they must take the risk of making their own choices.

In Perry's approach, learning requires the students to make sense of their own experiences. As the students grow and develop, they discover new and complex ways of thinking and seeing. He argued that this often demands a "loss of innocence" that may be painful and difficult: "It may be a great joy to discover a new and complex way of thinking and seeing; but yesterday one thought in simple ways, and hope and aspiration were embedded in those ways. Now that those ways are left behind, must hope be abandoned too" (Perry, 1981, p. 108).

He cautioned us that it takes time for students to come to terms with their new insights—"for the guts to catch up with such leaps of the mind" (Perry, 1981, p. 108). Time is needed to mourn the loss of simpler ways of thought. This need may explain why development is stepwise, rather than steady.

MENTORING

Mentors lead students along the journeys of their lives. They are trusted because they have been there before. According to Levinson (1978), mentors are especially important at the beginning of people's careers and at crucial turning points in their professional lives. Mentors have already accomplished the goals sought by the students. A mentor is typically an older, more experienced member of the profession who takes the student "under his or her wing." The role of the university as a parent substitute is reflected both in our reference to the university as our "alma mater" and in the term *in loco parentis*—in the place of the parent. In the beginning, the student often experiences the mentor as a powerful authority—a parental figure with almost magical skill.

This view is also a common source of trouble in the relationship, especially with students who have a long history of problems with authority figures. It is in the context of this relationship that students grow into their professional identity. In the early stages of their intellectual and personal development, students look to the mentor as all-knowing and expect to be given the right answers to questions. They are not ready to see the mentor's clay feet. As the students learn and develop, they recognize that authorities are not always right and that even their mentors are human. Eventually, with a growing sense of their own professional identity, students recognize mentors as colleagues.

Daloz (1986) provided a valuable framework for understanding the tasks of mentors. Effective mentors provide a balance of support and challenge (see Figure 9.1) and, at the same time, provide vision.

Support. "Be with" the students. Let them know they are understood and cared for. Such support promotes the basic trust needed to summon the courage to move ahead. The mentor is tangible proof that the journey can be made. Listen empathically: What is it like in the students' world; what gives it meaning; how do they view themselves; how do they decide among conflicting ideas; what do they expect from their teachers? Notice the similarities between these learner-centered questions and those we suggest that doctors ask of their patients to explore the illness experience (see Chapter 3 in this volume).

Challenge

		High	Low
Support	**High**	Growth	Confirmation
	Low	Retreat	Stasis

Figure 9.1. Framework of the Tasks of Mentors.

SOURCE: From *Effective Teaching and Mentoring: Realizing the Transformational Power of Adult Learning Experiences* (p. 214), by L. A. Daloz, 1986, San Francisco: Jossey-Bass. Copyright 1986, Jossey-Bass. Reprinted with permission.

Setting aside time indicates that students are important as people and that their ideas matter. "Preparatory empathy" is helpful. Before a student arrives, remind yourself what it was like to be a student starting a new rotation. Prepare yourself to respond to indirect cues. Students are generally wary at first and may not be direct with authority figures. Express positive expectations. Whenever possible, build self-esteem and confidence.

Challenge. "Assign mysterious tasks, introduce contradictory ideas, question tacit assumptions, or even risk damage to the relationship by refusing to answer questions. The function of the challenge is to open a gap between student and environment, a gap that creates tension in the student, calling out for closure" (Daloz, 1986, p. 213).

In setting tasks, the mentor brings learners to "see" a world they might not otherwise have observed. Examples of tasks are projects and reading assignments. The purpose may be clear or unclear. In the film *The Karate Kid*, the tasks set by Mr. Miyagi were not understood by the Karate Kid until he was ready to know. Asking pointed questions, pointing out contradictions, and offering alternative points of view may help push students past the stage of dualism; encouraging them to take a stand on a difficult issue or to criticize an expert may help them develop a commitment.

Engage in discussion. College learning involves the construction of new frames of meaning; therefore students need the opportunity to try out their understandings and to clarify contradictions. Hearing the views of their peers is often helpful.

Heat up dichotomies. Pushing different points of view and challenging students to comprehend the differences and to deeply appreciate contrasting points of view stimulate personal development.

Vision. Inspire learners to see new meaning in their work and to keep struggling despite confusion and discouragement. Vision sustains learners in their attempts to apprehend a fuller, more comprehensive image of the world.

One way of providing vision is through being a role model for the students. The film *Educating Rita* depicts an example of this. Rita's teacher represented the person she wished to become. The attraction was very powerful at first, almost like a love affair, each filling the other's needs. But as Rita grew and developed, she left her teacher behind. This example illustrates the power and potential danger of role modeling for both student and teacher.

Provide a framework for understanding the developmental tasks facing the individual student. Offer a vision of the physician's role that goes beyond the enumeration of skills to be learned and that acknowledges the personal and spiritual qualities inherent in becoming a healer.

Suggest a new language. Metaphors give us new ways to think about the world. The good teacher helps students not so much to solve problems as to see them anew. To think in new ways requires us to learn a new vocabulary and especially to develop new metaphors. Physicians may be constrained by the dominant military metaphor in medicine that implies we are always "doing battle" with disease and must adopt an aggressive, interventionist approach. To see physicians as "witnesses" to their patients' illnesses, who help give that suffering some meaning, frees physicians to be more imaginative in their approaches to healing (some of these are described in Chapter 5). For example, in *A Fortunate Man*, Berger (Berger & Mohr, 1967) described John Sassall, a country doctor working in a remote and impoverished English rural community:

> He does more than treat them when they are ill; he is the objective witness of their lives. . . . He keeps the records so that, from time to time,

they can consult them themselves. The most frequent opening to a conversation with him, if it is not a professional conversation, are the words "Do you remember when . . . ?" He represents them, becomes their objective (as opposed to subjective) memory, because he represents their lost possibility of understanding and relating to the outside world, and because he also represents some of what they know but cannot think. (p. 109)

It is the doctor's acceptance of what the patient tells him and the accuracy of his appreciation as he suggests how different parts of his life may fit together, it is this which then persuades the patient that he and the doctor and other men are comparable because whatever he says of himself or his fears or his fantasies seem to be at least as familiar to the doctor as to him. He is no longer an exception. He can be recognized. (p. 76)

THE NATURE OF CLINICAL PROBLEMS

Donald Schon (1983, 1987) provided valuable insights into the nature of clinical problem solving. Learning to be a physician is learning to recognize, analyze, and manage clinical problems. Common sense implies that the nature of these problems should influence the nature of medical education. Schon (1987) made a distinction between "the high ground" and "the swamp." In the high ground, patients present with problems at least partially defined. The clinician's task is to rule in or rule out a few clearly defined disease entities. If disease is identified, the standard therapy is prescribed; if no disease is found, the patient is reassured, with the expectation that he or she will be satisfied and so will not bother the physician again. In the swamp, where most clinicians work, the job is not so clear-cut. Much of the time, no disease can be identified to explain the patient's suffering; even when disease is found, there is often no effective treatment. Frequently, it is more helpful to explore what the patient is worried about and to provide understanding and support, even when diagnosis is possible.

How can we teach this technique? To deal with problems on the high ground, students are taught about basic science and how to apply basic science knowledge to defined clinical problems. But for the messy situations that clinicians manage, this approach often is not helpful. To learn how to handle these situations, students must jump in and try their best with the support and guidance of a skilled practitioner. Schon points out that professional training often involves an inherent paradox: Students can only learn to be professionals by doing, but they do not yet know how to do it and the task is too complex to describe fully in words. Consequently, the teacher cannot tell them exactly what it is they must do; the teacher functions more as a coach, helping them along each step of the way, guiding the students' eyes, hands, heads, and hearts in doing. The teacher will challenge students with such questions as What will you do now? Why? How? Did you notice that . . .? What happened when you . . .? For example, in teaching interviewing skills, the teacher can give rules of thumb regarding question style but needs to get the learner doing things and observing what happens and making sense of it. Sometimes, it is helpful for students to observe a teacher thinking aloud as he or she tries to make sense of a problem.

Meno described this paradox of learning in the dialogue of Plato named after him (Hamilton & Cairns, 1961):

> But how will you look for something when you don't in the least know what it is? How on earth are you going to set up something you don't know as the object of your search? To put it another way, even if you come right up against it, how will you know that what you have found is the thing you didn't know? (p. 363)

Inherent in this paradox of learning is the learners' dependence on the teacher. For example, to learn the patient-centered approach, students must give up their old ways of doing things and perhaps even their old ways of seeing things. The conventional clinical method, which gave them a sense of competence, autonomy, and security, will no longer suffice. In learning this approach, they must be willing to suspend their disbelief in the teacher's point of view. This suspension can make students too vulnerable, and the cost of dependency may be too high. Schon (1987) noted:

> As he willingly suspends disbelief, he also suspends autonomy—as though he were becoming a child again. In such a predicament, he is more or less vulnerable to anxiety. . . . If he is easily threatened by the temporary surrender of his sense of competence, then the risk of loss will seem difficult or even impossible. (p. 95)

According to Dewey, students cannot be taught what they need to know, but they can be coached:

> He has to see on his own behalf and in his own way the relations between means and methods employed and results achieved. Nobody else can see for him, and he can't see just by being "told," although *the right kind of telling* may guide his seeing and thus help him see what he needs to see. (Dewey, in Archambault, 1974, p. 151)

Guidelines for Teachers

- Help learners develop sufficient skill and comfort with the conventional clinical method to be ready to move ahead to the next phase of learning.
- Show examples during training. Even if they are unable to transcend the conventional medical model, the idea that there is more to medicine than diagnosis and treatment may become apparent and serve as a model for future learning. It is important for teachers to share their struggles and challenges, modeling the ability to learn from their experience.
- Help learners learn how to attend to what the patient wants to talk about and to realize that listening may be more therapeutic than any biomedical intervention.
- Help learners develop survival strategies to avoid becoming overwhelmed. For example, physicians need colleagues with whom they can discuss difficult or emotionally draining encounters with patients.
- Help learners to reflect on their experiences and to learn from them. This knowledge provides the tools for a lifetime of learning.
- Use the relationship between teacher and learner to demonstrate aspects of the patient-doctor relationship. Use the same caring and attention to the humanity of the learner that we expect the learner to demonstrate with patients.

Conclusion

Learning to be a patient-centered doctor challenges young physicians to develop their skills and, more important, themselves. The task can feel overwhelming at times and may awaken feelings of vulnerability and terror as students grapple at the growing edges of their abilities. Their teachers must be responsive to their struggles and address learners' needs and concerns. Teachers must model, in their behavior with students, the quality of interaction they expect students to demonstrate with patients.

We have woven several strands of educational thought that provide the fabric of the dialogue metaphor of education. Medical education is a "journey through a swamp" guided by wise mentors who are sensitive to the issues involved in human development. At the same time, teachers must be skilled in the use of a variety of teaching strategies illustrated by the transmission metaphor (e.g., able to teach specific interviewing and history-taking skills). Combining this repertoire of teaching methods into a seamless whole will provide the learning environment needed to foster the human dimensions of medical education. It is only in such a setting that the patient-centered method can be mastered.

10

Dealing With Common Difficulties in Learning and Teaching the Patient-Centered Method

W. WAYNE WESTON

JUDITH BELLE BROWN

Teaching and learning the patient-centered method is demanding for many reasons. Medical practice often seems arduous enough when limited to the diagnosis and treatment of disease; suggesting to doctors that they also must consider patients' perspectives of the illness experience and the social context in which patients live their lives may seem overwhelming. This is especially true for young doctors struggling to learn their craft. In this chapter, we elaborate on some of the common challenges faced by those who strive to learn or teach the patient-centered clinical method and provide examples to illustrate how these common difficulties may be overcome.

The Nature of Medical Practice

Several characteristics of practice pose difficulties for learning. Hippocrates (*The Aphorisms of Hippocrates*, 1982) commented on this 2,000 years ago in his aphorism: Life is short; art is long; opportunity fugitive; experience delusive; judgment difficult. The long hours, lack of sleep, and personally draining nature of patient care often leave students and practitioners exhausted and emotionally spent. Physicians in this condition may have little energy to invest in learning to be patient-centered. In the long run, we argue, patient-centered care is more rewarding for both doctors and patients. But when doctors are harried, they are tempted to focus narrowly on a patient's presenting complaint alone and to end the visit as quickly as possible by ignoring any other concerns the patient may have. When doctors appear rushed, patients may collude in this approach by keeping their worries to themselves. This suppression reinforces some physicians' beliefs that most patients are interested primarily in quick solutions.

Although undeniable time pressures occur in practice, sometimes doctors are caught up in "busy work" to avoid the emotional demands of practice. Without a commitment to continuing personal growth and self-awareness, physicians may evade confronting the reasons for their avoidance. The following case serves as an example.

CASE EXAMPLE

A first-year resident described his discomfort with the recent death of his patient. He found the experience painful because, in spending time with the patient, he had developed a relationship. Unlike the deaths of patients who had remained strangers, this patient's death touched him deeply. He almost wished he had not become attached and was ambivalent about allowing himself to become vulnerable again. This experience was a turning point in his education: The opportunity to discuss his feelings with his peers and teachers helped him accept his pain as a necessary part of his learning and growth. He realized that protecting himself from further painful experiences by avoiding close relationships with his patients would rob him of one of the most valued aspects of practice. He also recognized that his relationship with the patient was the most helpful element of his care.

Discomfort With
Relinquishing Power to Patients

In disease-centered interviews, doctors simplify their patients' problems by reducing them to disease categories. The focus is on the problem, not the person; the personal, social, and cultural contexts are not relevant to the physician's central mission of diagnosis and cure. Another way in which the interview can be simplified is for both doctor and patient to agree that the doctor is in charge. The roles of doctor and patient are clear and distinct: The doctor's task is to make a diagnosis and to tell the patient what to do to recover; the patient's job is to comply with the "doctor's orders." Patient-centered interviews may be more complicated. Doctors are not only looking for disease but also actively seeking to comprehend their patients' suffering; in addition, doctors are striving to involve their patients in the decisions about what should be done. Many physicians are reluctant to inquire about a patient's expectations, for fear the patient will ask for something they disagree with; they are uncomfortable with confrontation and saying no. Doctors tend to see such disagreements as win-lose situations, wherein one opinion must prevail, rather than as potential win-win situations, wherein the ideas of both may lead to a more creative solution. In this latter approach, the textbook answer may not be the best response under the special circumstances of the individual patient. It may be particularly difficult for young physicians still struggling to develop their self-confidence as professionals to share power with their patients. The following example illustrates some of the issues that lead to power struggles between doctor and patient and the resultant failure to find common ground.

CASE EXAMPLE

A 55-year-old woman returned for a follow-up visit for hypertension. This was the third visit in which her blood pressure was about 150/100, and the resident was eager to start medication. But the patient was unwilling to take pills "for the rest of my life." She was concerned about cost and side effects; she wondered whether her blood pressure could be brought under control in some other way. The resident's first reaction was to try harder to convince the patient to begin drug therapy, and he assailed her with facts and figures. But the harder he tried, the more the patient presented her concerns. Finally, exasperated, the resident wrote a prescription and urged her to get it filled. He concluded the visit with a warning that he would not be responsible for any problems she might encounter should she fail to comply. As the patient left the office, she felt misunderstood and chastised and did not fill the prescription. The resident also felt misunderstood and frustrated by the patient's potential noncompliance and shared his concerns with his supervisor. They quickly agreed that doctor and patient were not on the same wavelength regarding treatment and explored ways to find common ground. In the discussion with his supervisor, the resident recognized that, in his eagerness to treat the high blood pressure, he had failed to ascertain the patient's understanding of her problem and the proposed treatment.

Reluctantly, on the insistence of her family, the patient returned 3 months later to have her blood pressure rechecked. When the resident learned that the patient had not filled the prescription and found her pressure unchanged, he decided to try the approach suggested by his supervisor. Although both patient and doctor acknowledged that her elevated blood pressure was a problem, they had quite different ideas about management. Instead of admonishing her, the resident tried to understand her reservations about taking medication. She told him about her father's long history of hypertension and the many complications he suffered from drug therapy. She was determined that this would not happen to her. The resident acknowledged that her concerns were legitimate and engaged her in a discussion of various treatment options. They reached an agreement about the approach to therapy: aiming for a blood pressure below 140/90; using home blood pressure monitoring; starting with nonpharmacologic methods of treatment; adding drug therapy if nonpharmacologic methods failed to achieve the target pressure within 6 months; and monitoring carefully for adverse effects of medication. Although the resident wanted to achieve optimum blood pressure control sooner than this, he recognized that it was more important for his patient to take an active part in her own treatment. By sharing the decisions about treatment with the patient, the resident avoided another power struggle and involved her in an effective therapeutic alliance.

The Need for Self-Awareness

Doctors who explore patients' cues to personal problems quickly find themselves discussing intensely intimate issues. When confronted with serious illness, patients often wonder about its meaning for them and their families. For example, it may raise fundamental questions, such as Why me? or What will happen to my children if I die? Other patients may present with symptoms that reflect their concerns about their marriage or employment. These situations may trigger questions and feelings in the physicians' mind related to their own current relationships or to unresolved issues from their families of origin. As a result, young physicians, with little life experience, may be overwhelmed by their feelings and may retreat into the conventional medical model (refer to Chapter 2 in this book) for self-protection. In addition, physicians may form some patient relationships that unconsciously replicate troubled relationships from their past; without insight, the physicians are likely to become entangled in the same difficulties.

Because the patient-doctor relationship is so intensely personal, such difficulties are inevitable at times. Students and physicians need opportunities to develop self-awareness. These issues must be addressed with sensitivity by the teacher, taking into consideration the students' level of comfort in discussing their feelings. Often this discussion can be in a small group so that all students learn from each other's insights; but sometimes this technique may be too threatening or overwhelming. Opportunities for one-on-one discussion also need to be available. The following example describes a teaching intervention that promoted self-awareness.

CASE EXAMPLE

In a teaching practice, a resident stepped out of a patient interview to consult with his supervisor. This was the second time he had seen the patient for tension-type headaches. The 45-year-old executive was not improving and initiated this visit to ask for a CAT scan referral. The resident was frustrated and angry with what he described as an "abuse of the system." His attempt to persuade the patient that the test was unnecessary terminated in a heated disagreement. He thought his medical knowledge had been rejected and his professional credibility undermined. He needed to win this argument! The supervisor recognized her student's vulnerability and need for support. But, from previous experience with this patient, the supervisor understood that his request probably stemmed from the death of his uncle from a brain tumor 6 months earlier.

The teacher's task was to help the resident ventilate his feelings and then help him explore why he had fallen into a win-lose relationship with the patient. He needed to understand how both he and the patient had contributed to this impasse. Then he had to find a way to convert the struggle into a win-win outcome. The resident recognized that his recurrent conflict with authority figures led him to experience the patient's request for reassurance as a demand for an unnecessary test and a challenge of his medical competence. Instead of exploring the patient's fears, he reacted by defending himself. He dismissed the patient's request as unwarranted, and the fight was on. After realizing what had happened, the resident was able to return to the patient, acknowledge that they had reached an impasse, and ask whether they could begin again. This request culminated in an exploration of the patient's concerns and fears about the headaches. After a careful neurological examination and discussion about why a brain tumor was highly unlikely, the patient was prepared to consider other causes for his headaches.

Later, the resident sat down with the supervisor to discuss options for exploring his problem with authority figures. The supervisor's recognition of his vulnerability had prevented her from criticizing his error and engaging in a parallel struggle that would have replicated the student's difficulties with authority. Instead, her nonjudgmental stance encouraged the development of his self-awareness.

For the most part, as physicians mature in personal and clinical wisdom, they become more comfortable with the uncertainties of medicine and the complexities of their patients' problems. Ongoing self-reflection promotes a deepening understanding of the patient-physician relationship.

Overemphasis on the
Conventional Medical Model

Several features of medical education and professional socialization may interfere with learning an effective clinical approach to the familiar problems presented by patients. Medical training indoctrinates students to see patients' problems as derangements of the "body-machine" and to be concerned about missing some rare but deadly disease. As a result, most students and many physicians attempt to find a disease to explain each of their patients' complaints. This effort may result in overinvestigation, unnecessary referral, and overprescribing. Also, patients' personal concerns may receive little attention because physicians are concentrating their thought and energy on ferreting out pathology. This lack is not surprising because the majority of medical students' clinical experiences are in large, tertiary care hospitals where they are exposed to very seriously ill patients. They often are overworked and may have little time to do anything but tend to the grave physical needs of their patients.

In the absence of an alternative model, it is understandable that young physicians will use the framework they are most familiar with—the conventional medical model. Physicians, when stressed or overwhelmed by the problems of a patient, often will revert to a simplistic focus on conventional medical diagnosis even if they have learned and have used a more sophisticated and comprehensive patient-centered approach.

One of our students, in describing her struggle to use the patient-centered method, expressed her fears that she would be mandated to relinquish the conventional medical model altogether:

> I *want* to remember that stuff [textbook information], you know?! Not only did I work hard to learn it and to remember it for a short while, and it has helped me to fend off staffmen in the past, but even without the quizzing, it is a form of security, a teddy bear of sorts. Beyond that, sometimes it's a source of pride, of excitement, of fun, of conversation with colleagues, a worldly treasure. Yeah, I know it's a treasure moths will soon destroy (to coin a phrase), but meanwhile I am trying to live in a world that demands these things!

The conventional medical model has a long history of success, is highly respected in our culture, and allows physicians to remain comfortably distant from patients and their problems. Also, if doctors do their best (biomedically speaking) and their patients do not improve, the physicians need feel no blame. If patients do not comply with their doctors' orders, then the lack of improvement can be blamed on the patients.

Students and physicians need to learn a more appropriate model, one that incorporates the power of the conventional medical model but that is not constrained by its narrow focus on disease. Such a model cannot be learned all at once. Students may need to learn each component of the model separately, and they also require opportunities to practice integrating their skills into a unified whole.

Concentration on History Taking
Rather Than on Interviewing

Students in first-year medical school have little difficulty learning how to inquire about patients' ideas and expectations concerning their illnesses. As they progress through medical school, however, they become consumed by the task of making the right diagnoses, and their interviews become less patient centered (Barbee & Feldman, 1970; Cohen, 1985; Helfer, 1970; Preven et al., 1986). This may be a consequence of the emphasis on taking a thorough history of each disease and completing a comprehensive functional inquiry. Much less attention is given to open-ended exploration of a patient's thoughts and feelings. Without practice, most young doctors feel uncomfortable inquiring about patients' personal lives. Often, the concern is that a patient will become emotional and perhaps cry or show anger; they worry that they will open up a "can of worms" they will not be able to handle. Physicians' training tends to make them cautious about trying new approaches with a patient when they feel uncertain about the outcome; they are also reluctant to try unfamiliar techniques if they feel uncomfortable or awkward. The most common excuse given to avoid asking about patients' personal concerns is lack of time. But it is not efficient use of time to search for a disease that is not present or to ignore a major source of patients' distress, such as their fears or concerns.

Alternatively, when physicians are learning the patient-centered method, they mistakenly equate it with a "psychosocial functional inquiry." The following example typifies this common misunderstanding.

CASE EXAMPLE

When a patient presented with concerns about her severe sore throat and about how long she was going to be off school, the resident interrupted her story, "Wait, I need to get to know more about your personal situation. Where did you grow up? What was your childhood like? Was there much conflict in your family?" These questions would be very useful in the appropriate context, but in this case they seemed unconnected with the patient's practical concerns about receiving effective treatment and getting back to school as soon as possible. The physician needed to be sensitive to any cues about how this patient's home and school situation were related to her illness, but not to impose a psychosocial agenda where it did not apply.

We must beware of creating a false dichotomy between biological medicine (the "body") and psychosocial medicine (the "mind") or between the conventional medical model and the patient-centered model. The model we advocate includes the conventional medical model and integrates all of the determinants of health in its method.

Teacher Inexperience

It takes considerable experience, first as a doctor and then as a clinical teacher, before a physician can integrate secondhand information about patients to make good decisions. To make the task even more complex, teachers are trying to assess not only the patients' problems but also the learners' problems. To succeed at this endeavor, teachers must consider many factors at the same time. First are several questions about students: Did they establish a comfortable relationship with patients that allowed the patients to mention everything they had in mind? Did the students pick up on all of the important cues the patients gave? Did the students mention to the teacher all of their concerns about the patients, or did they avoid those topics that might have disclosed their own ignorance? What are the students' blind spots? Unless the teacher has prior knowledge of the students or has witnessed their conduct in actual interviews with patients, it may be difficult to answer many of these questions. It is important to establish a climate of acceptance in which students are not punished for admitting ignorance. Students need to know that the teacher is depending on the information they gather to make important management decisions; hence they must state where they are confused or uncertain so that the teacher can explore or double-check these areas.

Second are questions to be considered about the patients: What more information does the physician need to make a reasonable diagnosis? Why did the patient present now? What are the patient's thoughts, feelings, and expectations about the problem? Here, too, prior knowledge is invaluable. But unless teachers have seen the patient-student interactions, they must depend on obtaining second-hand information from students.

Third is the fact that inexperienced teachers may be concerned about their reputation among their students and may feel a need to prove themselves by demonstrating their excellence as clinicians. The dilemma for physicians teaching a patient-centered approach is that the value system of the medical school is often at odds with this approach. Excellence may be defined in terms of one's technical prowess and diagnostic acumen, but rarely in terms of one's ability to relate to patients. In teaching at the bedside, the discussion may focus on the latest drug for the patient's problem, rather than on exploring the patient's experience of the illness. For young students, desperate for unambiguous answers in the chaotic and messy domain of clinical medicine, knowing the latest drugs for various diseases is highly valued. They have not yet learned how to deal with uncertainty. Students may reward teachers who can provide black-and-white answers and may discount teachers who urge them to address not only the patient's disease but also the illness experience in the context of his or her life setting. Young students may feel overwhelmed by the complexity of clinical medicine and resent the teacher who appears to make their task more difficult. Thus students' needs for certainty and simplicity, coupled with the teacher's need for acceptance by peers, can have a powerful influence on novice teachers.

Competing Demands on Teachers

Teachers are pulled in many directions at once: They are expected to be exemplary role models and to see enough patients to earn a living; they must prove themselves credible among their academic colleagues by engaging in research and by publishing papers; they must add their fair share of teaching of both undergraduate and postgraduate students; and they must serve on the many committees and working groups of the university and professional associations that depend on their involvement. Faculty members increasingly are finding themselves stretched thin and forced to set priorities. Too often, time for teaching is cut back because there are fewer institu- tional rewards for these activities than for research or clinical care. Teaching the patient-centered approach may be time-consuming, con- sidering that teachers would want to observe student-patient interac- tions, to provide constructive feedback, and to adequately explore students' personal issues that may be evoked by the discussion.

Teacher Overprotectiveness

Including students in patient care changes the patient-doctor rela- tionship and creates several dilemmas for teachers. Clinical teaching makes the doctor's job more complicated; the teacher, in this context, is responsible not only for the quality of patient care but also for the quality of the student's learning experience. Sometimes, the two responsibilities seem to be at odds. Physician discomfort in these situations may interfere with student learning. Doctors may be more hesitant to allow students to practice on their patients than the pa- tients are themselves. For example, physicians may falsely assume that their patients would not want to discuss with a student their feelings about being ill. This assumption may be a reflection more of the physician's discomfort than of the patient's uneasiness. Most patients are willing to cooperate to benefit the students' learning, provided that the students are appropriately supervised and are not attempting something for which they are ill prepared.

11

Teaching the Patient-Centered Method

Instructional Methods

W. WAYNE WESTON

JUDITH BELLE BROWN

The setting for learning in a medical school is molded by many things, but the major artisan is the teacher whose work penetrates to unnumbered patients who profit or suffer from encounters with his or her students. This responsibility is too heavy for tradition, inertia, or ennui to be allowed to dictate the teacher's actions; as a scientist, he or she can do no less than prepare for this responsibility as carefully as he or she would prepare to be a physician or an investigator. The means are at hand. All the teacher need do is use them. (Miller, 1961, p. 296)

In this chapter, we describe the learner-centered approach, a conceptual framework for teaching that parallels the patient-centered clinical method. In addition, we discuss the relationship between learning objectives and teaching methods and illustrate these educational principles with applications to learning and teaching the patient-centered approach. The Appendix is a set of learning objectives that can serve as a guide for both teachers and learners.

143

Being Learner-Centered

In the same way that patient-doctor relationships have changed, so too have the relationships between learners and teachers. These parallels provide a framework for understanding the changing roles of teachers and learners in medical education. This framework also serves as a tool; learners' experiences of their relationships with their teachers help them understand their relationships with patients. For example, when teachers interact with learners as autonomous adults responsible for their own learning, they illustrate the kind of relationship teachers expect learners to develop with patients. Analogous to the patient-centered clinical method, the learner-centered method consists of six interactive components (see Table 11.1 and Figure 11.1):

1. Exploring learning needs and aspirations
2. Understanding the whole person
3. Finding common ground
4. Incorporating prior knowledge
5. Enhancing the teacher-learner relationship
6. Being realistic

EXPLORING LEARNING NEEDS AND ASPIRATIONS

In the learner-centered approach, teachers and learners collaborate in defining the objectives for learning on the basis of an assessment of both gaps in essential knowledge and students' areas of special interest. This approach shares many features with self-directed learning (Brookfield, 1985, 1986; Candy, 1991; Cheren, 1983; Knowles, 1980; Merriam, 1993; Mezirow, 1991; Tough, 1979) but also requires an active role on the part of the teacher. Cheren pointed out that self-direction in learning is not an all-or-none phenomenon, but rather is a continuum with *self-directed* at one end and *teacher-directed* at the other. He pointed out seven major aspects of a learning experience that can be expressed as a series of questions:

1. What is to be learned (both in general terms and specifically)?
2. How is the learning to be used?
3. How is the learning to be accomplished?
4. How is the learning to be consolidated, demonstrated, or shared?

TABLE 11.1 A Learner-Centered Model of Teaching

The Six Components of Teaching One-to-One

1. Exploring learning needs and aspirations
   A. Prescribed needs (the "official" curriculum, requirements for competence)
   B. Aspirations—felt needs (self-assessment, expectations, feelings, level of performance)

2. Understanding the whole person
   A. The "person" (life history and personal and cognitive development)
   B. The context (opportunities and constraints of the learning environment)

3. Finding common ground
   A. Priorities
   B. Teaching/learning methods
   C. Roles for teacher and learner

4. Incorporating prior knowledge
   A. Preexisting learning needs
   B. Strengths

5. Enhancing the teacher-learner relationship

6. Being realistic
   A. Time
   B. Team building

5. How and by whom is the learning to be assessed? (And what criteria are to be used to determine that a satisfactory or better level of learning has been achieved?)

6. How, if at all, is the learning to be documented?

7. What is the time limit, or schedule, for the effort? (Cheren, 1983, p. 26)

Learners who are completely self-directed will answer all of these questions on their own. But often this task is too daunting, especially for students unfamiliar with the content to be learned. "So much work is required to exercise complete control over every aspect of a learning project that it is not practical or worth the effort to try to exercise all that control all the time" (Cheren, 1983, p. 27). For these learners, the questions will need to be answered in consultation with their teachers. For many reasons, one should begin by determining students' deepest felt concerns about what matters most in their education. This determination enhances motivation (Forsyth & McMillan, 1991; Lucas, 1990; Spiegel, 1981) and personal responsibility for learning.

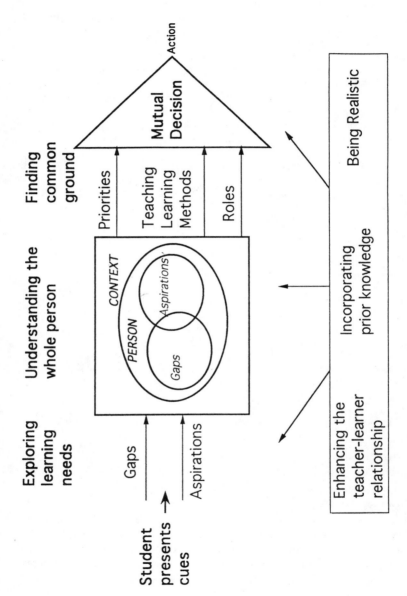

Figure 11.1. A Learner-Centered Model of Teaching.

Furthermore, it gives them practice in self-assessment, a critical skill for lifelong learning. But students may not be aware of all of the requirements for competent practice and may have blind spots regarding their own abilities. Addressing these issues is a paramount responsibility of their teachers, who must have a clear conception of the requirements for practice and the skill to assess students on each of these. In addition, teachers must be able to articulate these learning needs in a constructive and practical manner. Teachers help students understand what is important for practice, not by threatening them with difficult exams, but by providing opportunities to experience the need to know. Such motivating experiences can take many forms: stories of teachers' own struggles to learn, role play with simulated patients, seminars with previous students who discuss the evolution of their own understanding of their discipline, and discussion with patients about qualities they most admire in physicians.

UNDERSTANDING THE WHOLE PERSON

Akin to the two important dimensions of understanding the patient as a whole person (the patient's stage in his or her life cycle and the context) are two dimensions of understanding the student as a whole person: the student's educational stage of development and the learner's context.

In the same way that physicians oversimplify their patients' complex problems by focusing on the pathophysiology of disease, so too do teachers oversimplify their students' educational needs by concentrating on their major learning deficiencies. Teachers may speak of making a "learning diagnosis" in terms of the gaps in students' knowledge, skills, and attitudes, compared with the objectives of the program. This description may be very helpful, as far as it goes, but it may fail to convey an accurate understanding of what the learner as a person really needs. Students are different in so many important ways: in previous life experiences, courses taken, preferred learning styles, willingness to take risks, self-confidence, and resistance to change. Some students are fascinated by people and seem to interact comfortably with anyone; others are more at ease in the world of ideas and things. Even students from the same school and the same class have vastly differing abilities and learning needs. It is crucial to identify these so that the students are not put into situations where they are out of their depth. It is also essential to identify strengths so that valuable time is not wasted practicing skills already mastered while ignoring areas of deficiency. Students differ in their stages of personal, cognitive, and professional development (described in Chapter 9). Understanding these multiple differences will help teachers tailor learning activities to the specific qualities of each student and also will help them provide better advice to the student. For example, they can warn students about learning experiences that will be especially difficult or particularly valuable.

The learning environment strongly influences what can or will be learned. Armstrong (1977), in describing medical education, depicted the power of the curriculum to structure experience and thereby bring about implicit knowledge. The educational frame informs the student which common sense knowledge can be brought into medical school and what is not acceptable. Thus the hidden curriculum transmits certain beliefs and values to the student. The central concept that permeates the deep structure of the hidden curriculum is the notion of disease. This gives students the belief that they know what disease is while being unable to conceptualize it formally. Students learn to see the world as a dichotomy between those who have a disease and those who do not. The dilemma they face is that they have no categories to describe people who are ill but have no disease. The teachers' challenge is to confront the hidden curriculum by making it explicit and to help students consider alternative conceptual frameworks.

FINDING COMMON GROUND

Three elements are key in finding common ground in the learner-centered approach: (a) establishing priorities, (b) choosing appropriate teaching-learning methods, and (c) determining the roles of both teacher and learner.

Priorities. Difficulties arise when there is a conflict between what a student wants to learn and what a teacher wants to teach. When the official curriculum reflects the realities of practice, rather than is a difficult hurdle for students to jump in order to "prove themselves," such conflict is less likely. Also, students may become frustrated when so many objectives are required that no time is left to address topics of particular interest. A learner-centered approach does not hand over the curriculum to the students, but it does respect their intelligence, common sense, and good intentions by involving them in decisions about what to learn, when to learn it, how deeply to focus, and how to evaluate their learning.

Teaching and Learning Methods. Several studies defining the characteristics of excellent clinical teaching support the use of a learner-centered approach (Irby, 1978; Schwenk & Whitman, 1987). Whether done from the point of view of learners, teachers, or both, these studies agree that clinical teachers should demonstrate the following:

1. *Clinical competence* (including good skills, procedures, and patient-care abilities). Such teachers have a humanistic orientation, stressing the social and psychological aspects of patient care. They possess an excellent fund of knowledge and are able to present information in a clear and well-organized fashion. They are prepared to share with students their struggles and successes with patients as a model of continuing learning.

2. *Enthusiasm for teaching.* Such teachers obviously enjoy associating with students and make themselves accessible to them.

3. *Supervisory skills.* Such teachers are sensitive to patient and student needs simultaneously and involve students actively in patient care and in their own learning. They provide clear and appropriate direction and give frequent constructive feedback. Helpful feedback is the teacher's description of students' effective and ineffective behaviors that shows them how to improve their ineffective behaviors (see Table 11.2). They emphasize problem solving by challenging students to discuss their thinking processes and give students an opportunity to practice skills and procedures. They are open to criticism from students and use it to enhance mutual learning.

4. *Effective interpersonal skills.* Such teachers are sensitive to students' concerns, such as feelings of inadequacy, and demonstrate a genuine interest in students through a friendly manner. Whenever possible, they build the self-esteem of students. Hurst (1987) argued that the most important thing an effective teacher does is to form a good relationship with each student: "Students judge the quality of teaching by determining how much teachers give of themselves" (p. vii).

Roles of Student and Teacher. McKeachie's outline of teachers' roles helps us understand the many and varied responsibilities of teachers (McKeachie, 1978, pp. 68-82). On the one hand, teachers function as

TABLE 11.2 Characteristics of Effective Feedback

Feedback is descriptive, rather than evaluative—for example, "I noticed that you avoided eye contact with the patient when talking about sex." versus "You are rather weak in interviewing skills."

Feedback is specific, rather than general—for example, "You picked up well on the patient's back pain but seemed uncertain how to explore the patient's expectations about management." versus "You had better do some work on your clinical skills."

Feedback focuses on behavior, rather than on personality—for example, "Your infrequent use of silence and open-ended questions reduces the chances of the patient telling you what's on his mind." versus "You aren't interested enough in your patients."

Feedback involves sharing information, rather than giving advice. This encourages learners to decide for themselves how to handle the problem.

Feedback limits the amount of information to how much learners can use, rather than overloads them.

Feedback is verified or checked with learners—for example, "How do you feel the interview went?" versus "You were terrific!" Positive feedback may be confusing or unhelpful if students thought they really did a poor job.

Feedback pays attention to the consequences of feedback. The verbal and nonverbal responses of students are noted. Students are asked to comment on the feedback.

Feedback avoids collusion: It is not always essential to provide brutally frank feedback; this may be harmful. However, it is vital not to provide meaningless and misleading or dishonest feedback—for example, "That was okay," when it was really poorly done.

SOURCES: Berquist & Phillips, 1975; Casbergue, 1978; Ende, 1983; Westberg & Jason, 1991.

facilitator, ego ideal, and person; they support and encourage students by the force of their own personalities. Students incorporate aspects of their teachers into their own developing professional identities and often form close personal relationships with them. On the other hand, teachers are experts, formal authorities, and socializing agents; they are guardians of the traditions of the profession and stand as trustees who decide whether each student measures up for admission into the ranks. In this sense, no matter what else they represent in the minds of their students, they are powerful and sometimes intimidating authority figures. Thus teachers wear many hats and have complex multidimensional relationships with their students.

INCORPORATING PRIOR KNOWLEDGE

Previous knowledge of learners' strengths, weaknesses, and special interests accelerates the learning process and increases the intensity and complexity of the knowledge, skills, and attitudes to be mastered. The curriculum can be viewed as a spiral: The same content may be encountered on several occasions, but each time it is assimilated in greater depth. Pacing is also important. When students become overwhelmed by the emotional intensity of a learning experience, they may need a break. Then, restored, they return to the learning environment ready to proceed with the next learning task. For example, helping dying patients come to terms with their mortality is often psychologically draining, and students may need an emotional respite. This may happen only with the support and permission of their teachers. Finally, continuity allows the whole process to be more efficient and effective. The important personal and contextual issues, so critical in determining what will be learned, cannot be communicated easily from one teacher to another.

ENHANCING THE LEARNER-TEACHER RELATIONSHIP

Above all else, the relationship between teachers and learners is the single most important variable affecting the outcomes of learning. Good teachers have a desire to help others learn that transcends the problems that teaching creates. Teaching interferes with physicians' intimate one-on-one relationships with their patients. It slows them down. It exposes their weaknesses and areas of ignorance. It demands a positive regard for the learners even when their behavior may frustrate or upset the teacher. Congruence between the patient-centered method and the process of teaching it is essential. For example, just as our commitment as doctors is to the person and not the disease, so too our commitment as teachers is to the learners and not to the subject matter. This commitment transcends individual learning problems or specific skills to be learned. It extends into the very being of the learners and challenges them to stretch themselves to their limits. Such learning may require students to experience painful self-discovery or to make difficult personal changes. Students often defend against such self-awareness and may find themselves in conflict with their teachers over the need for change. At this stage in the development of their professional identities, they often experience ambivalent feelings about their teachers: On the one hand, they wish for a dependent relationship in which their obligations are spelled out and clearly limited; on the other hand, they resent the imposition of control and long for independent responsibility. Their feelings may vacillate from one extreme to another, depending on the complexity and volume of patient care, fatigue, and feelings of self-efficacy. It is not surprising that intense emotions may develop in the student-teacher relationship, replicating similar feelings with other powerful authority figures from the students' past. Working through this transference may enhance the students' self-understanding and prevent similar reactions from occurring in the future. It requires the development of an intimate and trust-based relationship before such intensely personal learning and growth can occur.

Supervision of psychotherapists shares many similarities with clinical teaching, especially regarding the importance of the relationship between teacher and learner. Alonso (1985) summarizes this aspect:

> The development of a clinician from novice to expert is primarily an emotional, maturational process, much like the development of a child from infancy to adulthood. . . . It is assumed that a transference relationship will develop between therapist and supervisor and that this transferential field will become a primary vehicle for influencing the student's clinical growth. . . . There is a concerted effort to shore up and strengthen the supervisee's healthiest defences, either by reducing the ambiguity or by helping the trainee to tolerate the inevitable confusion of clinical work. . . . When difficulty occurs . . . this regression is seen as a healthy and expectable rite of passage. . . . In fact, the clinician who never regresses in the course of training is probably avoiding the more difficult levels of learning that occur in the unconscious merger of patient/ therapist and may be keeping too great a distance between self and patient. (pp. 47-48)

A number of teacher behaviors contribute to the creation of an impasse with learners: the need to be admired, the need to rescue, the need to be in control, the need for competition, the need to be loved, the need to work through unresolved prior conflict in the supervisor's own training experience, spillover from stress in the personal or professional life of the supervisor, and tension between supervisor and the administration of the institution (Alonso, 1985, pp. 83-104). This list highlights the paramount importance of a healthy and open relationship between teachers and learners, characterized by empathy, genuineness, and positive regard (Rogers, 1951). It is one of the very special privileges of teaching to share in the struggles of students for growth and self-actualization.

BEING REALISTIC

Teachers must recognize that they cannot be all things to all people. The destructive myth of faculty members as "triple threats" (Mundy, 1991), expected to be exemplary clinicians, outstanding researchers, and superb teachers, casts faculty into impossible situations of role overload. Not only is this behavior self-destructive, but it also demonstrates poor role modeling for students. As a consequence, students may set unachievable objectives for themselves. Conversely, to avoid replication of their teachers' lifestyles and to prevent role strain, students may impose inappropriate limitations on the responsibilities they will assume. One outcome of the establishment of rigid boundaries between their personal and professional lives is lost opportunities for learning and growth—for example, working in settings where the hours of work are limited, interactions are superficial, and all complex problems are referred (e.g., walk-in centers); limiting hours of practice or range of services provided (e.g., refusal to provide home visits, hospital visits, or palliative care). The patient-centered clinical method requires doctors to become involved in the full range of problems their patients present but acknowledges the importance of setting reasonable limits on how much time and energy will be expended. Although more effective time management will ease some of the problem, the answer is not that simple. Each doctor must discover how to juggle competing demands while maintaining an openness to both patient needs and personal and family needs. Thus it is important for teachers to strike a balance for themselves and to create a learning environment in which students can discover how to be realistic.

An important feature of modern medical practice is teamwork. Students need opportunities to work in effective multidisciplinary teams and to collaborate with other health care professionals. They need to learn how to be effective team members and team leaders. Doctors traditionally have seen themselves as team leaders and have been reluctant to learn from other health care professionals. This "medical chauvinism" is anachronistic and counterproductive. Young doctors in training have an opportunity to complement their traditional medical education by learning from teachers in other health disciplines. Team teaching is a powerful method for faculty members to model collaborative teaching and learning. Another valuable way in which medical students learn about the roles and functions of other professionals is by sharing learning experiences with students from other health care disciplines.

Principles of Teaching and Learning

In this section, we outline the relationship between learning objectives and teaching methods. Learning objectives are of several varieties, and each has specific conditions to facilitate learning (Gagne, 1977; Gagne & Briggs, 1979; Haney, 1971). For example, learning a new concept, such as the distinction between disease and illness, requires a much different educational experience from learning a skill, such as responding with empathy. Thus it is important for teachers and learners to recognize these differences between the types of learning in planning any instructional event. Because a learner-centered approach requires collaboration between teacher and student, it is important for both teachers and students to be conversant with these distinctions.

Verbal Information. This consists of ideas, propositions, and "facts"— the basic alphabet of knowledge. Without knowing the names of things, it is difficult to communicate with others in the field or to learn more complex knowledge. For example, the terminology used in the patient-centered model of practice provides teachers and learners with a common vocabulary for discussion. Much of this material can be learned effectively from lectures and reading and benefits from repetition.

Intellectual Skills. These are discriminations, concepts, and rules— the ability to interact with the environment by using symbols. Individuals possessing intellectual skills have a sufficient understanding of a body of knowledge for elucidating principles and identifying novel examples of concepts. For example, the student will be able to discuss the four dimensions of patients' illness experiences—ideas, expectations, feelings, and effects on function—and be able to recognize each element in his or her encounters with patients.

This type of learning is facilitated by stimulating recall of previously related knowledge and by guiding the new learning via a statement, question, or cue. Concepts "discovered" in this manner, as compared with being learned in a lecture, are more accessible to learners when they need to retrieve the concept in a new situation. Providing occasions for learners to perform their newly learned skill in connection with a new example is invaluable.

Problem-Solving Skills. These are the abilities to use verbal information and intellectual skills to deal with a situation that is novel to the learner at that point in time. Problem solving is a complex process that includes the capability to recognize the problem, skill in generating alternative solutions, and judgment in selecting an appropriate option. Attitudes relating to the content of the problem, self-confidence, and comfort with uncertainty all greatly influence the learner's ability to deal with a specific problem at a specific time (Haney, 1971). Prerequisite intellectual skills and verbal information are needed to solve specific problems. For example, when students are learning to reach mutual agreement with patients regarding treatment, it is useful for teachers to remind them about the three aspects of finding common ground—problems, goals, and roles. This reminder will be of particular importance when learners find themselves disagreeing with their patients about one or more of these aspects. Learners will need the skills to recognize when these prerequisites are missing and should be able to seek them out appropriately. There is no substitute for practice using problem-solving skills in a variety of novel situations.

Psychomotor Skills. These are the abilities to coordinate muscle movements in a smooth, regular, and precisely timed fashion (e.g., using body language and communication skills). Students need to know what the skills look like. Written educational objectives or a description of the skills may help, but a demonstration is even more helpful, especially for novices. Students need to learn each of the "part" skills and also the order in which each part is performed. Learning is facilitated by repeated practice in a situation that provides feedback. Feedback is absolutely essential to effective learning of psychomotor skills. The nature of the feedback should be varied, depending on the skill level of the learner. Novices will need fairly detailed and specific feedback about their performance: what was done well and what needs more practice or additional skill. As learners improve and develop a clearer idea of what a good performance looks like, they become more aware of their own shortcomings. At this stage, they need guidance to improve specific, discrete skills and practice putting them all together.

It is important to distinguish between application and acquisition practice. *Acquisition practice* occurs when a student is first learning a skill. It is useful at this stage of learning to practice one component of a skill at a time and to do it over and over again. Simulated patients are useful for this type of practice, but even real patients can be used. Students can be asked to concentrate on a specific part of the patient-centered method (e.g., determining patients' ideas and expectations about the visit). *Application practice* is done to consolidate learning of part skills in a coordinated and integrated manner, similar to the manner in which the skills will be used in the application setting. It is important to recognize students' levels of skill. They should not be expected to perform a complex communication skill on a real patient—for example, breaking bad news—if they have not had an opportunity to practice the essential part skills first—for example, empathy and support. Coaching is also vital; learners need someone to provide continuing feedback and moral support in the setting in which they will apply their new skills.

In learning a new skill, students typically go through four stages as they develop from novices into mature professionals (see Figure 11.2). The respective roles of teacher and student change as the student becomes more skilled. In the *stages of initial awareness* and *awkward use*, the teacher is the expert; the task is to define objectives, demonstrate the skill, guide the student, provide feedback, and evaluate the student's performance. The student's task is to follow instructions.

In the *stage of conscious application*, the teacher is a facilitator who suggests alternatives, negotiates objectives, and shares evaluation with the learner. The student's task is to select appropriate alternatives and to share in the evaluation.

In the *stage of natural integration*, the teacher is a consultant who provides feedback. The student's task is to define his or her own objectives and evaluate his or her own performance.

Attitudes. These are internal states that influence the choices of personal action made by individuals—predispositions to approach or avoid a situation. A number of attitudes have been identified as important for effective practice—for example, a willingness to become involved in the full range of difficulties that patients bring to their

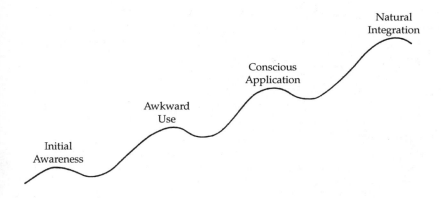

Figure 11.2. Stages of Skill Learning.
SOURCE: From "Increasing Awareness and Communication Skills," by S. Miller, D. Wackman, E. Nunnaly, and P. Miller, in *Connecting Skills Workbook*, 1989, p. 2. Littleton, CO: Interpersonal Communication Programs, Inc. Reprinted with permission.

doctors, and not just their physical problems. Attitudes may be learned from an emotionally toned experience following a course of action. For example, while a doctor was conducting a routine cervical smear, he uncovered a history of brutal childhood sexual abuse. Following self-disclosure of her story, the patient began to weep and then sobbed uncontrollably for some time. The doctor was overwhelmed by the patient's story and felt anguished and helpless. From that point on, he was extremely reluctant to inquire about the sexual histories of his female patients. Another example is the joy and sense of connectedness experienced by physicians at the time of a normal delivery, reinforcing their acceptance of the disruption in personal and practice schedules.

Attitudes are learned also from models—admired or respected individuals. All of us have an unconscious tendency to model ourselves after our heroes. This is a very potent teaching tool in the medical setting, where there is often prolonged and intimate one-on-one contact between teacher and student. Unfortunately, modeling is largely unconscious, and students may pick up their teachers' foibles, as well as strengths. Specific teaching methods can be used also to facilitate the learning of attitudes: discussion groups, mentoring, one-on-one supervision, videotape review of patient encounters (Premi,

1991), Balint groups (Balint, 1957; Brock, 1986; Maoz, Rabinbowitz, Hertz, Katz, & Hava, 1992), sharing genograms (Crouch, 1986), and discussion of the classic and modern literature about the human condition. These educational interventions may be insufficient to meet the needs of some students and physicians; if difficulties with patients become pervasive or chronic, personal therapy is required.

To summarize, the needs of the learner and the tasks of the teacher will vary with the desired learning outcome (Gagne, 1977). Facts are learned effectively from books and lectures; principles are learned by struggling with the material and applying it to new examples; problem solving is best learned by trying to solve problems in a variety of situations; psychomotor skills are learned by practice in situations that provide feedback; and attitudes usually are learned by interacting with respected models. Hence, teachers must be prepared to fill many roles: resource person, facilitator of learning, manager of learning resources, provider of feedback, and role model.

Learning Objectives

The Appendix describes each of the six interacting components of the patient-centered clinical method and outlines the knowledge, skills, and attitudes needed by physicians practicing this approach. In planning any learning experience, it is important for students to know where they are going (their objectives); otherwise, they may end up somewhere else (Mager, 1968, 1984). Most lists of objectives are either so short and vague that they are not helpful to the novice or so long and detailed that no one reads them. We have tried to avoid both extremes, to produce a usable list, by linking the educational objectives to the components of the medical interview. In this way, the curriculum is rooted in doctors' everyday interactions with their patients. But no list of objectives can stand alone. It is our hope that students and teachers will use this list as a focus for joint discussion and for the development of learning plans. The list can be used also for evaluation by learners assessing their own learning needs and by teachers providing constructive feedback. This list is not intended to be exhaustive, but rather to focus on what is most important. Objectives regarding the physician's conventional role are mentioned only briefly, not because they are less important, but because most readers already will be familiar with them.

12

Teaching
the Patient-Centered Method

Practical Tips

W. WAYNE WESTON

JUDITH BELLE BROWN

I n the previous chapters on teaching, we described the parallel processes of patient-centered and learner-centered approaches; we explored the human dimensions of learning; and we addressed many of the difficulties in learning the skills of patient-centered care. In this chapter, we focus on some of the practical issues involved in teaching patient-centered medicine.

Structural Issues

The context of learning is crucial. Students are unlikely to learn patient-centered medicine in an environment where it is not practiced or from teachers who do not value the principles underlying the method. Likewise, effective teaching is more apt to occur in a setting that supports and rewards it. Several issues about teachers need to be considered:

Interest and Skill in Teaching. Not all faculty members like teaching; some are more interested in administration or research. Academic units should be set up so that faculty members can focus on what they most value, and not be forced to spend too much time on activities for which they have no aptitude.

Faculty "Reward System." Faculty should be promoted on the basis of excellence in one or two areas of academic work and not be expected to be all things to all people. In many universities, teaching and patient care often are undervalued; faculty who devote most of their energies to these areas may jeopardize their careers. This possibility creates a conflict of interest: Spend more time with their patients and students, or commit more time to academic areas, such as research, that are rewarded by promotion and tenure. Teaching and practice must be seen as scholarly activities in their own right (Boyer, 1990).

Opportunities for Faculty Development. Teachers are made, not born. Without training in teaching, medical faculty tend to emulate previous medical school teachers. Often, this means copying less effective approaches. Many faculty members are interested in teaching but find it difficult or frustrating because they have had no preparation for the job. All faculties of medicine need a well-planned program of faculty development with a special emphasis on helping new faculty members learn their academic craft. Faculty members often are selected for their skills in research, administration, or teaching. Their reputations as clinicians are considered, but their clinical skills are rarely assessed in a rigorous manner. As a result, some faculty members will need additional training to improve their skills in using a patient-centered approach. Even faculty who are intuitively patient-centered will need opportunities to learn the theoretical basis of the model and to master the techniques to pass these skills on to their students. It is very difficult to teach the patient-centered method in an environment that does not enthusiastically embrace the approach or that fails to acknowledge the need for ongoing development and renewal.

Time. A central challenge for academe is to find a way to restore the sacred idleness so necessary for contemplation. Without time for thinking, teachers end up going through the motions, following algorithms or recipes that often are unproven. Good teaching takes time—to establish intimate relationships and to challenge the status quo by searching the literature for better answers. Learning the patient-centered method also requires time for observation and feedback.

Several important aspects of the practice setting also need to be considered:

Setting. Tertiary care teaching hospitals are becoming less and less appropriate sites for learning about relationships and communication with patients. Patients either are being admitted for day surgery or are so sick that they can barely converse with the doctor. It is almost impossible to develop long-term relationships with these patients. Alternative settings that are more conducive to learning the patient-centered method include physicians' offices in the community, patients' homes, chronic care facilities, and palliative care settings.

Clinicians are busy and not always available when students are scheduled to arrive. Consequently, effective teamwork is needed. Much of the teaching falls on the shoulders of the residents, nurses, and other members of the professional team who usually are given no preparation for the task. They may be unaware of the objectives for the students and may be asked to evaluate them without being provided any guidelines. They rarely are given advice about how to teach. As a minimum, all members of the professional team should be aware of:

when students are to arrive

the objectives for the students' experience

the evaluation system for the students

the role of students on the team and the level of responsibility expected of them

any special tasks or assignments expected to be completed by the students

the patient-centered model and the various methods used to teach it in that setting

Patients. Students and physicians learning patient-centered medicine need opportunities to work with patients of both sexes, all ages, many cultures, and with a vast range of problems. Patients also need to be given adequate preparation for and explanation of the students' roles and responsibilities.

Physical Plant. Space must be adequate for students to be integrated into the setting; they need a place to put their personal belongings, as well as a comfortable work space. In ambulatory settings, sufficient examining rooms are needed for students to see patients on their own without interfering with patient flow. Space for private discussions about patients or about students' concerns is essential.

It is impossible to teach the patient-centered method without providing constructive feedback to students. Effective feedback requires repeated direct observation of the student interacting with patients. Opportunities for observation, either with one-way mirrors or videotape, is invaluable. Videotape review, in particular, provides a powerful opportunity for enhancing self-awareness. Even without such equipment, it is possible to observe student-patient interactions directly by sitting quietly in a corner of the examining room. But, it is often difficult for the teacher to avoid being drawn into the interaction and quickly taking over.

Common Teaching Methods

Several common teaching methods, depending on their application, may be very effective or, at worst, destructive to student learning (see Table 12.1). Great teachers throughout the ages have used parables—stories with a message—to instruct and inspire their students. "War stories" may be entertaining and even instructive, but often they are told to enhance the reputation of the teller. A crucial distinction rests in the purpose of the narrative—whether to brag or to teach.

Using a one-on-one interaction with a student to give a lecture misses out on the major advantages of clinical teaching. Learning is directly proportional to the learner's degree of involvement.

A common distortion of the Socratic method is "Guess what I'm thinking!" Rather than probing and questioning learners to help them deepen their own understanding, the teacher asks leading questions or gives hints to help students guess the right answer. One hazard of this approach is that students stop thinking for themselves and, instead, start second-guessing the teacher. Some teachers think that being Socratic means never answering students' questions. Often,

TABLE 12.1 Comparing Common Teaching Methods

Less effective	More effective
"War stories"	Parables
Mini-lectures	Dialogue
"Guess what I'm thinking!"	Guided discovery
"Put down"	Critique the behavior, not the person
Never answering the question	Sometimes answering the question
Grilling	Challenging

teachers like this will turn every student question back on the student: "What do you think about that?" or "Why don't you look that up tonight and tell me tomorrow what you learned." Used appropriately, these techniques are invaluable, but sometimes students are so confused or overwhelmed that they need more help. Sometimes the answers they seek are not in the books; sometimes, especially in an ambulatory care setting, the student needs immediate advice to help a waiting patient. Sometimes, when teachers never answer students' questions, they begin to think they do not know any of the answers, and their credibility and effectiveness as teachers are lost. Answering students' questions too often, however, may foster dependence and convey the message that students are not capable of learning for themselves.

One of the most destructive acts a teacher can commit is to "put down" a student; students rarely forgive such behavior and will not respect a teacher who does not show respect for them. Students may learn facts from a teacher they do not like, but they will not heed the teacher's principles or values. It is especially dangerous for teachers to put down one student in front of others; they then lose the respect and credibility of the whole group of students.

Although drill may be appropriate for memorizing the dosages of emergency drugs, grilling—putting a student "on the hot seat"—is usually inappropriate. Those who advocate its use argue that it helps toughen up students and prepares them to keep cool in the stressful situations of clinical practice, where they must think and act quickly.

In its typical form, grilling involves repeated questioning of one student until he or she gives a wrong answer or gives up by confessing that he or she does not know the answer. The teacher moves on to other students and continues the process until all have been shown inferior to the teacher. This approach is said to motivate students to try harder but usually ends up in a game of clinical one-upmanship, and the focus is often on esoteric or trivial information. This approach may encourage competition, rather than teamwork, teaches that not knowing is "bad," and may leave students feeling put down. It is difficult for students to develop comfortable relationships with teachers who use this approach excessively. The vast majority of students in medicine are motivated to work hard. Excessive pressure from the teacher not only is unnecessary but also may be counterproductive. An overanxious student does not learn well. In a supportive environment where teachers demonstrate a genuine interest in the people they teach, students generally blossom and put forth their best efforts. In such a setting, teachers can challenge students' conclusions or even their basic assumptions without provoking so much defensiveness that the students cannot learn. An effective challenge preserves, and may even enhance, the learner's self-esteem.

Each of these teaching methods illustrates the distinction between teacher-directed and learner-centered approaches to education as described in Chapter 11. The more effective methods, described in Table 12.1, all focus on the needs of the learner more than on the interests of the teacher and are rooted in a fundamental respect for the learner.

Tips on Clinical Supervision

1. First clarify the patient's situation and the major problems to be addressed.
2. Ask the patient's name. In settings where patients are well known, the teacher will have a vast store of knowledge about previous illnesses, life experiences, and typical responses to stress. Knowing which patient the student is discussing will often generate key hypotheses about the current situation. This process models the importance of continuity of care and the value of the patient-physician relationship.
3. Avoid premature conclusions. One of the hazards of familiarity is the danger of drawing conclusions before fully exploring all possibilities

of the current situation. It is often useful to brainstorm—consider all options without the constraints of what is probable or practical.

4. Refrain from being the fountain of all knowledge. It is important for students to take ownership of their own learning and to relate the current clinical situation to their own experiences.

5. Ask students to "think aloud." Such thinking will often reveal to them where they are stuck.

6. Provide a conceptual framework. Decision trees and diagrams are helpful to organize masses of data or to uncover gaps in information. Use the chalkboard for clarification. When students are confused or unclear about a patient's problem, it is often useful to depict the situation as shown in Figure 12.1. In these situations, it is common to have a large mass of data about the patient's diseases and even some ideas about the patient's illness experience. But often, the sections on "Person" and "Context" are sparse. This visual representation helps the students recognize the deficiencies in their understanding of the patient and suggests areas for further inquiry. The diagram can be used also to document the accumulating knowledge about the patient. When a student is having difficulty working with a patient, the source of trouble often is related to finding common ground. Figure 12.2 illustrates a useful grid for identifying disagreements between patient and physician regarding management. In our experience, difficult interactions are reflected by differences of opinion about the nature of the problem, the goals of treatment, and the roles of patient and doctor in management. Filling in the grid makes the conflict obvious and leads naturally into a discussion about how to deal with their differences.

7. When students reach the limits of their knowledge, ask how they are going to seek more understanding of the issues. Schedule a definite time to follow up on what they learn.

8. When the decision cannot wait, offer a suggestion. If possible, offer options and encourage students to choose from them and to explain their choices.

9. Use questions to clarify what students are saying, rather than to probe their ignorance.

10. Use chart review; it is particularly helpful for assessing the strength of the evidence for the student's diagnostic conclusions and proposed investigation and management. The traditional record needs to be modified to fit the patient-centered method. For example, students should include information about the patient's "illness experience" (ideas, feelings, expectations, and effects on function).

11. Provide videotape review; it is vital for helping students examine their own reasoning process. The tape stimulates recall of their thought

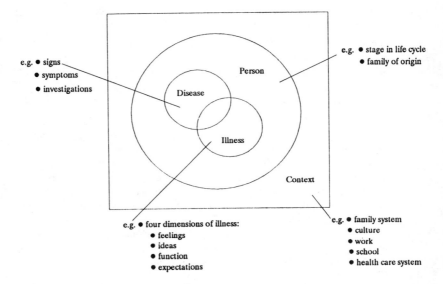

Figure 12.1. Understanding the Whole Person.

processes during the interview and can be used to challenge them about why they asked certain questions, why they ignored others, and why they did not ask questions that were on their minds.

12. Role play with simulated patients to offer students the possibility to practice in a safe situation and to try different approaches to the same situation. The opportunity to stop for a time-out is valuable for reflecting on the interaction and to receive feedback from the "patient," teacher, and other observers. This technique is also helpful in learning how to manage clinical situations that are uncommon and that may not present themselves to every student.

13. Prepare students to focus on specific behaviors and then give them an opportunity to discuss their observations. Learning from role models should not be a passive activity. For example, before the teacher and student enter the examining room, it is helpful for the teacher to explain what he or she will be attempting. If the student already has seen the patient but has been unable to determine the patient's experience of illness, the teacher may remind the student about the four dimensions that need to be explored and briefly outline the kinds of questions that could be asked. After the encounter, they will discuss the student's observations and the teacher's reasons for certain actions.

Issue	Patient	Doctor
Problems		
Goals		
Roles		

Figure 12.2. Finding Common Ground.

Conclusion

In this chapter, we highlighted a number of practical guidelines for teaching the patient-centered method. Effective teaching and learning require an environment that provides the necessary resources: patients, time, and space. It also must reward faculty for contributing their energies to becoming exemplary role models and clinical supervisors. It may be possible to teach some of the elements of the patient-centered method in the absence of this infrastructure, but without it, success is limited.

13

The Case Report
as a Teaching Tool for
Patient-Centered Communication

THOMAS R. FREEMAN

This chapter presents a potentially powerful tool for teaching patient-centered concepts: the patient-centered case presentation (PCCP). The chapter begins with a review of the evolution of case presentation approaches, presents the patient-centered case presentation with an example, and concludes with an assessment of the advantages of such an approach.

Review of
Case Presentation Approaches

The traditional format of the case presentation that evolved during the time of Sir William Osler was recognized very early as a valuable tool in the teaching of medicine (Cannon, 1900). It generally begins with a brief description of the patient, followed by the history of the present illness. Next comes past history, family history, patient profile, and examination findings. Investigative results, such as laboratory work, X-rays, pathology reports, problem list, and management plan,

AUTHOR'S NOTE: Parts of this chapter were published previously in *Family Practice: An International Journal, 11*(2), 1994.

usually round out the presentation. This form of presentation accurately reflects the conventional clinical method that is based on the biomedical model (McWhinney, 1988).

The written medical record was greatly improved by the method of L. L. Weed (1969), and his problem-oriented medical record has been widely accepted. This method made problems the organizing principle of the record and separated subjective and objective components. This form of written record has had a great influence on the format of oral case presentations, as well.

The biopsychosocial model proposed by Engel (1977) was an attempt to apply systems theory to clinical problems. This model, along with the recognition that psychological and social factors play a role in illness events, led to the inclusion of these topics in many case presentations.

The conventional case history or report has been criticized for being heavily dependent on scientific language that, although seemingly precise, leaves much of reality aside (Schwartz & Wiggins, 1985). Abstract scientific language excludes the human, lived experience of patients and obscures the fact that where illnesses are unique, disease labels are classificatory terms only (McCullough, 1989). This problem is as true of chronic illness as it is of acute illness (Gerhardt, 1990). By minimizing the importance of the patient's story and subjective experience, the conventional case history separates biological processes from the person (depersonalization) and minimizes the physician's role in producing findings or observations (Donnelly, 1986). This form of presentation is primarily doctor and disease centered. "The message is clear, disease counts; the human experience of illness does not" (Donnelly, 1986, p. 88).

Hawkins (1986) advocates a method she calls the "clinical biography," in which the scientific and humanistic are complementary, each representing different attitudes to the human experience. She points out that case history and biography are similar in that they involve a lot of interpretation and are to be understood in the "context" of the narrative.

From a phenomenological perspective, the clinical encounter can be viewed as a hermeneutical exercise involving the interpretation of multiple "texts." Such a hermeneutic model poses a number of questions, the most important being, "How can the ill person, both as text and co-interpreter, be restored to centrality in the clinical encounter?" (Leder, 1990).

Efforts to change the focus of case histories to include more accurate descriptions of patients as persons are as diverse as the elegant literary work of Luria (Hawkins, 1986) and Sacks (1986) and the innovative and pragmatic teaching methods of Donnelly (1989) and Charon (1986).

Donnelly (1989) suggests that the human aspects of medicine can be addressed by teaching stories (which pay attention to what has happened in the interior world), instead of chronicles (which stick simply to a recitation of events). He asked housestaff to include in the history one or two sentences about what the patient's understanding of the illness was and how it affects his or her life in an effort to help the physician empathize more accurately.

Charon (1986) states that the physician's effectiveness increases with empathy and teaches the "empathic stance" by asking medical students to write stories about their patients. These stories are considered to be adjuncts to the hospital chart and do not replace the traditional case write-ups. Charon suggests that the students are molded into the kind of doctor their teachers want by becoming the kind of writer their teachers want (Charon, 1989).

The need remains for a further elaboration of these techniques in the teaching of students and housestaff. Basic changes have to occur in the way medicine is taught.

Anspach (1988) points out that the presentation of case histories is an important part of the medical training of students, interns, and residents. Usually given before an audience of peers and senior medical people, these presentations are important both for their content and as part of the socialization process. They are a powerful way of teaching and reinforcing a particular worldview. With the evolution of the clinical method, it is an appropriate time for a change in the way case histories are presented to more accurately reflect and reinforce the new method and the worldview on which it is based.

Description of
Patient-Centered Case Presentation

In a sharp departure from the conventional case report that focuses on the organic pathology of the patient, the patient-centered case presentation (PCCP) gives primacy to the patient and the total experience of the illness and associated pathology. Unlike the conventional method, in which "the objective truths of medicine are recorded in the 'language of abstraction' " and are not "related to the existence of the individual" (Wulff, Pedersen, & Rosenberg, 1986, p. 132), the PCCP regards objective truth as of less interest when it is not related to the individual.

The PCCP focuses on an "acquaintance with particulars" (McWhinney, 1989a). It begins with a description of the particulars of the case under study and then proceeds to a discussion of the general (other cases or studies that may share similar features). There may be a discussion of a single case or several cases that seem to express a common theme.

The PCCP, by going from the particular to the general and from the subjective to the objective and back again, performs a cycle that ultimately informs the presenter with a greater understanding of the patient.

Table 13.1 is a comparison of the conventional case presentation and the patient-centered case presentation; how the items of information of the conventional approach are incorporated into the PCCP is highlighted.

The Patient's Chief Concern or Request. This portion of the presentation consists of a brief statement of the symptomatology, as well as the illness behavior (McWhinney, 1972) that brought the patient to the encounter. It should address the patient's actual reason for coming.

The Patient's Illness Experience. A description of the experience of the illness should include some quotations from the patient that particularly illustrate the subjective quality of the illness. For example, when discussing an individual for whom pain is a predominant feature, it would be appropriate to include the pain descriptors the patient used in communicating the discomfort. Metaphors are particularly helpful here because they are linguistic structures that bear epistemological weight (Carter, 1989; Donnelly, 1989). Knowing the metaphors that patients use to describe their illness gives the clinician greater insight, understanding, and empathy. The language for the metaphoric landscape is "not found in traditional textbooks of medicine, but in articulate memoirs of illness, insightful fiction, poetry, drama and the examined experience of our own illnesses and those of our family and friends" (Donnelly, 1989, pp. 134-135). As in the patient-centered clinical method, the patient's feelings, ideas, expectations, and the effects

TABLE 13.1 Comparison of Conventional and Patient-Centered Case
Presentation

Conventional case presentation	Patient-centered case presentation
1. Chief complaint	1. Patient's chief concern or request
2. History of present illness	2. Patient's illness experience; quotes from the patient; feelings, ideas, expectations, effects on function, meaning of illness
3. Past medical history medication, allergies, observations	3. Disease – History of present illness – Past medical history – Review of systems – Physical exam – Laboratory, etc.
4. Family history	4. Person – Patient profile – Individual life cycle phase
5. Patient profile	5. Context – Family history – Genogram – Family life cycle phase

6. Review of systems	6. Patient-doctor relationship (The clinical encounter) The dyad itself
	– Transference/countertransference issues
	– Finding common ground
	  – Problems
	  – Roles
	  – Goals

7. Physical exam	7. Assessment (problem list)
8. Laboratory database	8. General discussion Illness experience—Literature (pathographies, poetry); medical literature (clinical epidemiology, pathophysiology, other case reports, medical anthropology)
9. Problem list	9. Proposed management plan
10. General assessment	
11. Proposed plan	

of the illness on function are mentioned here, including the meaning of the symptoms to the patient.

Observations. The observation portion of the presentation involves the disease, person, and context dimensions shown in the diagram that presented an overview of the patient-centered clinical model (Figure 2.1 in Chapter 2). This section is subdivided into observations about the disease, including the standard elements of the medical history (history of present illness, past medical history, review of systems, physical exam, and relevant laboratory work), issues related to the person (patient profile, life cycle phase), and context (family, job, environment).

The Patient-Doctor Relationship (Clinical Encounter). This portion involves a discussion of not only the technical management issues (e.g., drug and nondrug therapies) but also how the patient-doctor dyad can be developed into a healing relationship (Cassell, 1985a). Issues of self-awareness, feelings about the patient, and struggles to make effective connections are appropriate, as are any issues related to finding common ground between the doctor's agenda and the patient's agenda (see Chapter 5 for a detailed description of finding common ground and Chapter 7 for more on enhancing the relationship).

Assessment (Problem List). This portion involves summarizing the issues that need further assessment or intervention in any of the four areas of person, disease, illness, or context.

General Discussion. Having discussed the particulars of the case, the presentation then turns to the general issues raised by the case. The issues selected for discussion are chosen by the presenter from elements of the case that he or she found most interesting or puzzling. In this way, the case helps instruct the presenter. General issues can be grouped into those related to the experience of the illness and those related to pathophysiology, epidemiology, sociology, and medical anthropology.

First-person accounts of the experience of illnesses are becoming more common. Literature and poetry provide many examples of individuals who have written in a lucid and illuminating way of their personal experience of an illness (Broyard, 1992; Cousins, 1979; Frank, 1991; Mukand, 1990; Styron 1990). Indeed, this type of writing has recently undergone a resurgence (Hawkins, 1993), and an acquaintance with it will provide the presenter with improved insights into the way the illness is affecting the patient. It will be necessary for faculty to accumulate a usable bibliography of such material as it appears not only in journals but also in newspapers, magazines, and books (Baker, 1985). In addition, the movie industry has focused on this area, and occasionally a short video can very effectively communicate the trials of a particular sickness.

This section of the PCCP includes a discussion of any relevant medical literature pertaining to the case. It should incorporate the current understanding of any pathology or clinical epidemiology (prevalence, natural history, the sensitivity and specificity and predictive value of any tests, and effects of intervention).

This portion also involves a knowledge of the published scientific literature concerning the disturbed psychological and social functions that have been observed in other individuals with similar problems.

Proposed Management Plan. This portion of the presentation is an opportunity to use the information gleaned from the discussion of the general issues and to integrate this knowledge into a management plan.

An Example

The following example of a PCCP is derived from the author's practice. The numbers in the headings correspond to the numbered patient-centered case presentation items shown in Table 13.1. The presentation begins with a description of the particulars of this case and is followed by an outline of some of the general issues raised by the case. Many of these issues were identified by residents when this case was presented to them. In a full case presentation, it is expected that the presenter will choose one or more of the issues to discuss in detail. The particular issues chosen should be decided by the presenter and reflect that person's learning needs. I have italicized key words in the patient's discourse that he used repeatedly to describe his understanding of the situation.

1. THE PATIENT'S CHIEF CONCERN/REQUEST

Brian (a pseudonym), 26 years old, attended the office because he had become more interested in doing something about his *lifestyle*. This interest was precipitated by recent laser surgery for treatment of diabetic retinopathy. As a result of the laser treatment, his vision had become more blurry, leading to some difficulty reading and causing him to rethink what was going on with his life.

2. THE PATIENT'S ILLNESS EXPERIENCE

To a great extent, Brian's illness experience revolved around his feelings and ideas about diabetes and the meaning, to him, of this label. When asked about the personal meaning of diabetes, he replied:

> . . . a change in lifestyle . . . your life has to be more routine . . . eating . . . exercise . . . you have to *control* eating, *control* your insulin. At one point, it [diabetes] was running my life; I wavered from letting it run my life to wanting to make it a very minimal part; now, I'm trying to find a *balance* between a routine and not letting it run my life.

His greatest fear developed after receiving laser treatments, when his vision became blurred: "Oh my God, I'm going to go blind!" Some of this blurring had resolved. He had since learned that, to a certain extent, this was to be expected after laser treatments. He expressed some anger at not being warned of the side effect of the procedure. He understood that the blurring may have been related also to *control* of his blood sugar. Even though some of the blurring had cleared, it forced him to consider some of the long-term consequences of diabetes: "My vision could become bad enough that I couldn't read." This fear took on even greater dimensions in view of his recent decision to become a teacher. The consequences of his recent treatments made it necessary that he sit at the front of the classroom. He denied that this change was a concern, but one sensed that this denial was wearing thin, as evidenced by the fact of his attendance to the office at this time.

3. OBSERVATIONS (DISEASE)

History of Present Illness. Brian was diagnosed with insulin-dependent diabetes mellitus at age 11. He had been on varying doses of insulin since that time. Several episodes of hypoglycemia occurred in his early adolescence.

His experience with visual difficulties was the most recent reminder of diabetes. When this first developed, he was new to the city and attended a walk-in clinic; he subsequently was referred to an ophthalmologist.

Past Medical History. Aside from his diabetes, Brian's past medical history was without significant events. There had been no surgery. There were no known drug allergies.

Current medications: Insulin-Lente 15 units, Crystalline 15 units in a.m., Lente 20 units, Crystalline 15 units in p.m. He only occasionally checked his blood sugars with a glucometer at home when he thought it was particularly high (he associated this with feeling "sluggish": "In my mind, I visualize my *blood getting thicker*"). He was evasive when pressed about what levels of glucose he was finding at these times but finally recalled numbers in the 300s or 400s on the "old scale."

Review of Systems. Aside from some persistent blurred vision, ROS revealed only occasional intestinal gas every 3 or 4 months.

Physical Exam. Brian presented himself in a detached manner. Even when talking about his fear of blindness, he talked in a monotone. He was clearly articulate and intelligent but left you with the impression that he distanced himself from his feelings as much as possible. He declined being weighed but appeared to be 10 to 15 pounds overweight. BP 126/82. Examination of the optic fundi revealed numerous microaneurysms but no hemorrhages. He declined any further examination at that time.

4. PERSON

During the past 15 years, Brian's experience and understanding of the disease had undergone some changes. As a child, his mother was deeply involved with the treatment of his diabetes. This involvement was not without its problems. He stated that when it was time for him to leave home and go to the university, one of the best parts was that his mother would not be there to *control* his diabetes.

He came to this city to start his university education and was involved in a program that emphasized tight control and careful monitoring of diet and exercise. Brian believed this approach was consistent with other parts of his life at the time, in that he could keep fairly consistent hours. After he finished his undergraduate education, however, his life became less controlled and predictable and so did his diabetic control. He found that close control interfered with his *lifestyle;* he thought he needed more spontaneity in his life, and routine was not consistent with this. This view coincided with frequent moves and an uncertainty about where he was going in his career. He let go of routine, and his lifestyle became scattered. He did the minimum required to manage his diabetic condition—took his insulin and watched his diet—but exercise and rest were ignored.

Brian described himself as an optimistic person. He said he bored easily and this was why he had gone through a period of frequent changes, although he thought that presently he was fairly settled. Recently, he had married a social worker who had taken a job with a local social agency. Brian felt more settled in terms of his career and his personal life. He thought things were "on track." Being married provided more routine. He started teachers' college this past fall.

Brian viewed himself as a lot like both of his parents. "I want to deny that I'm like my father but . . ." He believed he shared with his father the orientation that "my motivation comes from inside me. I know that I should look at external factors, but I don't. He's organized, and so am I." Like his father, Brian sometimes liked to be alone.

5. CONTEXT

Brian's family of origin consisted of his parents and two sisters. His older sister developed hydrocephalus and epilepsy, both of which were under control. She currently worked for the board of education in a neighboring city. His younger sister was alive and well. His father was 56 years old and had been diagnosed as having hypertension and circulatory problems. He had "several times been close to a heart attack." Brian attributed this to his father's "self-imposed stress. . . . He isn't very social, and he doesn't get much exercise. I think that's contributing to his problem." His mother was 55 years old and basically healthy, although she used to be overweight.

6. THE PATIENT-DOCTOR RELATIONSHIP

"I don't like people helping me. I'm really strong about that." Brian was unable to think of any way his doctor could be of help to him except for "routine medical problems." This clearly excluded helping manage his diabetes, as he made clear that that would be too much like his mother and he refused to let that type of relationship develop again. This refusal suggested some developmental and some transference issues.

He did not comply with a request to have some basic blood work done, although he took a laboratory requisition with him. He was invited several times to return for a complete physical assessment or simply to talk but so far has not done so, continuing to attend for minor episodic problems. To date, common ground has not been found, and agreement on the goals and priorities has not been reached.

7. ASSESSMENT (PROBLEM LIST)

1. Insulin-dependent diabetes mellitus
2. Diabetic retinopathy/threatened visual loss
3. Unresolved family-of-origin issues
4. Questionable compliance with diabetic regimen
5. Failure to find common ground about management

8. GENERAL DISCUSSION

In an oral case presentation, it is expected that the presenter fully discuss at least one of the issues raised in this section. The others may be outlined.

The Experience of the Illness. Two prominent issues are suggested by this case with respect to the experience of the illness: control and the fear of visual loss.

The potential or actual loss of control is a characteristic of most illnesses, whether acute or chronic. It is essential that physicians recognize the centrality of loss of control to any state of illness. Part of the physician's role as a healer is to restore a sense of control to the patient (Cassell, 1985a).

Compelling accounts of what it means to be blind or to face the imminent loss of vision are common in literature and poetry (Longhurst & Grant, 1989). Occasionally, in the lay press, appear eloquent first-person descriptions of individuals struggling with the fallout of diabetes (Fields, 1990).

A familiarity with such material will serve to inform the physician tending to Brian and to deepen his or her understanding of the subjective aspects of this man's illness. It may help the physician to provide advice on the day-to-day coping with the problems caused by the illness.

The Observations. From the standpoint of the biomedical model, some of the issues this case raises are euglycemia and diabetic retinopathy, the use of laser technology in treating such retinopathy, and the common sequelae of this procedure.

Under the rubric of "contextual issues" could be considered the family and the child with chronic disease (Battle, 1975; Leichtman, 1975).

Many of the life phase issues that Brian is facing are related to late adolescence. Consideration of the adolescent coping with chronic illness, therefore, would be appropriate here (Wolfish & McLean, 1974). The developmental tasks of identity and the capacity to form intimate relationships may be thwarted by an excessive preoccupation with illness and the sick role.

The Patient-Doctor Relationship. Stein (1985a, Chap. 3) argues convincingly for physician awareness of the unconscious communications taking place between patient and doctor that influence the illness/disease process. One of the cases he reports ("The Contest for Control: A Case of Diabetes Mellitus in Multiple Contexts") is an excellent introduction to consideration of the relationship issues with patients such as Brian.

9. PROPOSED MANAGEMENT

In a situation such as the one developed with Brian, it is clear that common ground has not yet been defined. It becomes necessary for the physician to go back and find common ground with the patient on each of the three areas: problem definition, goal setting, and roles.

TABLE 13.2 Finding Common Ground With Brian About Management

	Doctor	*Patient*
Problem	Diabetes mellitus Poor compliance Complications	Diabetes mellitus Interference with lifestyle
Goals	Better glucose control	Fewer symptoms Less interference with lifestyle
Roles	Provide information Gentle challenge but avoid paternalism	Independence Self-control

As Brian enters the early adulthood phase of his life, it will be particularly important that his physician develop a collegial relationship and avoid an authoritarian one that would echo the type of relationship he experienced with his mother and that he has spent at least the last 6 years trying to escape. The management can be summarized as in Table 13.2.

In a formal case presentation, therefore, a presenter could choose to expand on any one of the identified topics (the issue of control in illness experience, fear of visual loss, euglycemia and diabetic retinopathy, laser treatment of diabetic retinopathy and sequelae of treatment, the family and child with chronic disease, adolescence and chronic disease, and transference/countertransference issues). A review of such topics will help more fully inform the development of a management plan.

In using this method of case presentation with residents, my experience has been that there is a tendency to avoid topics around illness experience. This avoidance is best dealt with by stating the issue in the beginning, when the method is first presented, and by meeting with the learner/presenter at least 1 week before the presentation to review the proposed case and to direct him or her to the appropriate resources.

Advantages of the New Method

Case presentations can be viewed as "highly conventionalized linguistic rituals" that serve to socialize physicians in training to a particular worldview (Anspach, 1988). The PCCP, by placing the patient at the core of the presentation, reinforces the primacy of the person, rather than of the disease, without excluding the process of clinical decision making. In this way, it can serve to inculcate a more humane form of medicine and reinforce the basic values inherent in the patient-centered clinical model. It does this without sacrificing the more conventional type of information found in the standard case presentation.

In most medical schools, learning is largely passive (lectures) in the initial years. This method gradually gives way to the less structured format experienced in clinical rotations and residency training, in which the learner is expected to take a more active part in learning. It is not an unusual experience, after starting into practice, to feel somewhat at a loss about how to continue to be well informed. The rapid expansion of medical knowledge makes it impossible for any individual to always be completely up to date. Therefore, it is necessary that the graduate family physician have a method for continuing medical education that takes into account one's individual learning needs. Most experienced family physicians acknowledge that their most demanding teachers are ultimately their patients. The PCCP offers a format that can serve as a bridge between the passive learning of medical school and the active learning of medical practice. It recognizes the role of the patient in teaching us what we most need to know.

The usual reasons for making a case report are (a) a unique case, (b) a case of unexpected association, and (c) a case of unexpected events (Morris, 1991). The philosophy of the PCCP is that each case is unique and may, and often will, involve the unexpected. The only necessary motivation for undertaking a PCCP is a desire to come to a deeper understanding of the patient.

Summary

The patient-centered clinical presentation suggests a new way of presenting case material in medicine that is consistent with new clinical methods. Its proponents recognize that case presentations are an important part of the socialization of training physicians. By giving primacy to the subjective aspects of illness, this form of presentation reinforces an attitude of patient-centeredness.

This way of presenting a case forms a useful bridge between the passive and detached learning characteristic of much of undergraduate medical training and the active, personal learning required of a practicing physician.

PART THREE

Research on Patient-Centered Communication

14

Studies of Health Outcomes and Patient-Centered Communication

MOIRA STEWART

What is the rigorous scientific evidence that patient-centered communication with patients makes any difference to the patient or to the health care system? This chapter provides a review of research evaluating the impact of communication on patients' health. The chapter follows the conventional format of a formal literature review, beginning with the magnitude of problems in communication, then turning to the positive impact of communication, and then ending with a discussion. This review of previous studies sets the stage for the following chapters, which focus on current methods and projects, and leads us to think about where research should go from here. As clinicians considering ways to improve ourselves and as teachers setting priorities, we must consider the question: How worthy of our attention is patient-doctor communication?

This question has two sides: One considers the evidence of the magnitude of problems in communication; the other considers the evidence of the positive effects of communication.

Problems in Communication

Evidence suggests that a wide range of problems in communication are quite common. These problems include misdiagnosis: approximately two thirds of psychosocial and psychiatric problems are missed (Goldberg & Blackwell, 1970); 54% of patient complaints are not elicited by physicians; 45% of patient concerns are not elicited (Stewart et al., 1979); and on 50% of visits the patient and doctor do not agree on the nature of the main presenting problem (Starfield et al., 1981). One reason for such problems might be that physicians interrupt patients 18 seconds, on average, into the patients' description of the presenting problem (Frankel & Beckman, 1989). As well, patients complain about lack of information provided to them; for example, 83% of people believe in patients' right to information (Haug & Lavin, 1983).

Problems have been identified not only by studies but also from the general population, whose complaints to licensing bodies are frequently due to communication breakdowns (Munn, 1990). As well, negative headlines indicate the dimensions of the dissatisfaction—for example, "All Too Often, Communicating Is Not a Doctor's Strong Point" (Coleman, 1991); "Urgent Need for MD's to Relate Better to Patient" (Murray, 1991); and "Cold Hard Death, Cold Hard Doctors" (Davis-Barron, 1992).

Positive Effects of Communication

Of the many studies of the effect of communication, some used patient satisfaction as the outcome and have been reviewed elsewhere (Roter & Hall, 1992). Other studies associated communication with patient compliance (Sackett & Haynes, 1976). The 21 studies reviewed here considered patient health outcomes. They took place in a variety of medical settings, making their findings relevant to surgeons, anesthesiologists, internists, obstetricians/gynecologists, pediatricians, family physicians, and psychiatrists.

The following paragraphs as well as Table 14.1 present a brief summary of results of a literature review conducted by the author in 1994. In the 10 observational studies and the 11 randomized controlled trials (RCTs) reviewed in this chapter, communication was classified into two broad components: communication relevant to the traditional history-taking segment of the visit, which in this book is referred to as "exploring the illness experience"; and communication relevant to the management segment of the visit, which in this book is called "finding common ground." Studies in which communication was described in a way that could not be classified as exploring the

TABLE 14.1 Tabulation of the Components of Communication Studied by the Results

	Component of communication studied				
Result	Exploring the illness experience (EIE)	Finding common ground (FCG)	Both EIE and FCG	Other	Total
Positive results	2	8	5	1	16
Negative results	0	0	1	3	4
Inconclusive results	0	1	0	0	1
TOTAL	2	9	6	4	21

illness experience or finding common ground were categorized separately.

Regarding the component of exploring the patient's illness experience, eight studies related this component of a patient-physician encounter to health outcomes (two of this component alone, and six of this component in combination with other components). Four where RCTs, all of which showed positive results (Evans, Kiellerup, Stanley, Burrows, & Sweet, 1987; Greenfield, Kaplan, & Ware, 1985; Kaplan, Greenfield, & Ware, 1989a; Roter & Hall, 1991); four were observational studies, three showing positive results (Haezen-Klemens & Lapinska, 1984; Headache Study Group, 1986; Orth, Stiles, Scherwitz, Hennrikus, & Vallbona, 1987), and one showing negative (nonsignificant) results (Putnam, Stiles, Jacob, & James, 1985).

Two of the interventions were education programs for physicians: one aimed at increasing physician knowledge of history-taking and compliance-improving strategies (Evans et al., 1987), and the second about the emotional and diagnostic dimensions of the illness experience aimed at improving communication knowledge and skills (Roter & Hall, 1991). Physicians were taught to encourage patient talk, to avoid interruptions, to ask about the patients' complaints, to probe for concerns, to ask for the patients' understanding of the problem, to explore expectations, to explore the impact of symptoms on their lives, to ask for feelings, to compliment patient effort, to show empathy, and to show support. Two studies were conducted by the same team of investigators that designed an intervention for patients (Greenfield et al., 1985; Kaplan et al., 1989a). The intervention with patients sought to increase their participation in the interview with the physician by providing information about their own problem and care and by coaching them on question asking and negotiating skills. Although the intervention's explicit goals applied more to finding common ground than to exploring the illness experience, it is mentioned here because, in these two studies, the intervention succeeded in increasing the patients' statements about feelings, opinions, and information, clearly a part of exploring the illness experience.

The following dimensions of exploring the illness experience were identified as effective by three observational studies: (a) patients' perception that their problem had been fully discussed with the physician (Headache Study Group, 1986), (b) high use by physicians of many questions and emotional support (Haezen-Klemens & Lapinska, 1984), and (c) high degree of patient exposition during the history-taking segment—that is, patients giving information in their own words, not merely responding with yes/no answers (Orth et al., 1987). A second study of patient exposition showed no significant association with health (Putnam et al., 1985).

Communication between patients and physicians about the management/treatment plan been called "gaining compliance," "a negotiation process," and more recently, "finding common ground." Of the 21 studies reviewed, 15 related this component of the patient-physician interaction to patient health outcomes (9 of this component alone, and 6 of this component in combination with other components). Seven were RCTs, all with positive findings; and eight were observational studies—six with positive results, one with a negative result, and one with an inconclusive result.

Four interventions affected only finding common ground. All of these interventions were for patients, not physicians. Two were patient information programs, one by anesthetists about the expected nature of postoperative pain (Egbert, Battit, Welch, & Bartlett, 1964), and the other by taped messages describing radiation treatment and its effects (Johnson, Nail, Lauver, King, & Keys, 1988). The other two focused on encouraging patients to ask more questions in order to gain the knowledge they thought they needed to care for their condition (Thompson, Nanni, & Schwankovsky, 1990). One study revealed that the relevant communication improvements resulting from the intervention were (a) an increase in patients' asking questions and giving direction and (b) an increase in patients' effectiveness in obtaining information (Greenfield et al., 1988).

The important aspects of finding common ground in the observational studies were physicians' simultaneously providing information and emotional support (Haezen-Klemens & Lapinska, 1984); the physician giving objective information about the illness, tests, treatment, and side effects (Orth et al., 1987); information packages to patients (Rainey, 1985); use of surgeons who allow their patients a choice in their surgery (Fallowfield, Hall, Maguire, & Baum, 1990); and agreement of the patient and physician about the nature of the problem and the need for follow-up (Bass et al., 1986; Starfield et al., 1981). Two studies showed nonsignificant associations with health outcomes of an actual choice given to the breast cancer patients regarding the type of surgery be done (Fallowfield et al., 1990; Morris & Ingham, 1988). As well, one observational study found a positive relationship of explanation with recall and satisfaction, but not with health (Putnam et al., 1985).

Other components of communication have been assessed by three RCTs (Savage & Armstrong, 1990; Thomas, 1978, 1987) and one observational study (Hulka, Kupper, Cassel, Mayo, 1975).

Effectiveness of Patient-Centered Components

The effective aspects of exploring the illness experience were the physician asking questions particularly about the patients' complaints, concerns, understanding of the problem, expectations, impact, and feelings; the physician showing support and empathy; the patients being involved by expressing themselves completely; and the patients perceiving that a full discussion of the problem had taken place.

The effective aspects of finding common ground were patients asking more questions and being successful at getting the information they needed; information programs/packages for patients; physician use of information with support; physician willingness to share decision making with the patients; and agreement between patient and physician about the nature of the problem and need for follow-up.

This literature review of studies of health outcomes has clarified what aspects of the patient-centered approach have been well studied (finding common ground with 15 investigations), moderately well studied (the illness experience with 8 investigations), little studied (the relationship or the physician as therapeutic agent with 1 study), and not at all studied (achieving an integrated understanding of the whole person, prevention, and being realistic).

The bottom line "so what?" question has been answered with a convincing 16 studies showing positive results and 5 showing negative or inconclusive results.

The best studied components of the patient-centered approach can now be described on the basis of their known effective dimensions. One is heartened to see that the clinically derived theory on exploring the illness experience (described in Chapter 3) shows remarkable overlap with the dimensions revealed in this review, including exploration of patients' symptoms, expectations, ideas, feelings, and impact on function.

Similarly, the key clinically derived dimensions of finding common ground (described in Chapter 5) have been supported by the research reviewed. The studies demonstrated our four key dimensions to be effective: clear information; questions by patients; willingness to share (discuss) decisions; and agreement between patient and doctor about the problem and the plan.

15

Methods of Scoring Patient-Centeredness

MOIRA STEWART

The preceding chapter presented a review of studies of communication and health. Researchers used a variety of approaches to assess communication. This chapter is a brief review of the measures that are relevant to patient-centered concepts. As well, we present a reliable measure of Components 1 to 3 of the patient-centered approach described in Chapters 3, 4, and 5 of this book. The reader interested in research measures or in tools for educational evaluation will find a variety of approaches to choose from. Our intent is to provide a description, rather than a critical review of the measures. This chapter focuses on scoring methods from the quantitative tradition. Readers interested in qualitative approaches are referred to Chapter 16.

In general, the measurement approaches can be classed into four types: (a) those based on coding all statements made by patients and physicians, (b) checklists of physician behaviors, (c) rating scales, and (d) questions asked of patients and physicians after the encounter.

Coding

Coding approaches of verbal behavior of patients and physicians have been reviewed elsewhere (Stiles & Putnam, 1989). Coding is a frequently used approach in outcomes research (Bales, 1950; Greenfield et al., 1988; Kaplan et al., 1989a; Korsch, Gozzi, & Francis, 1968; Roter, 1977; Stiles, 1986), and although it has been used in educational evaluation, it usually is considered too time-consuming for such uses. The four best known applications of this approach are Roter's Interaction Analysis System, which uses 35 categories to code and then creates proportional scores of behaviors relevant to patient-centeredness (Roter, 1977); Kaplan and Greenfield's coding, which has been used to create patient-effectiveness scores, affect/opinion scores, and others germane to patient-centered concepts (Kaplan et al., 1989a); Stiles's Verbal Response Mode system, which codes both process and intent and creates proportional scores on patient exposition and physician explanation (Stiles, 1986; Stiles, Putnam, Wolf, & James, 1979); and Callahan and Bertakis's Davis Observation Code assesses the presence of 20 behaviors, focusing on content (e.g., chatting, history taking, health education) during each 15-second interval of an audio- or videotape (Bertakis & Callahan, 1992; Callahan & Bertakis, 1991).

Checklists of Physician Behaviors

Checklists are very common tools in educational settings but less widely used in research because very few checklists have been rigorously tested for reliability and validity. Two relevant and tested checklists are those of Blanchard, Ruckdeschel, Fletcher, and Blanchard (1986), whose interdisciplinary team of researchers and clinicians (medical oncology, social work, and psychology) created a 35-item checklist; and of Kraan, Crijnen, Zuidweg, Vander Vleuten, and Imbos (1989) and Kraan and Crijnen (1987), representing a wide variety of medical disciplines, who developed the 68-item Maastricht History Taking and Advice Checklist.

Rating Scales

Rating scales are common in educational settings. Some focus on skills, such as Stillman's (1977) 24-item Interview Rating Scale (which uses a 5-point scale for each item). Semantic differential scales focus on overall qualities, such as *organized ... disorganized* (Heaton & Kurtz, 1991) or affective quality of the encounter (Roter, 1977). Visual analog scales have been used to assess global performance (Blanchard et al.,

TABLE 15.1 Consultation Rating Scale

Please evaluate the consultation you have just seen by rating it on the following scales. Place a mark in such a position along each line to show how much you agree with each statement.

1. Nature and history of problems adequately defined	....	Nature and history of problems defined inadequately
2. Aetiology of problems adequately defined	....	Aetiology defined inadequately
3. Patient's ideas explored adequately and appropriately	....	Ideas explored inadequately or inappropriately
4. Patient's concerns explored adequately and appropriately	....	Concerns explored inadequately or inappropriately
5. Patient's expectations explored adequately and appropriately	....	Expectations explored inadequately or inappropriately
6. Effects of problems explored adequately and appropriately	....	Effects of problems explored inadequately or inappropriately
7. Continuing problems considered	....	Continuing problems not considered
8. At risk factors considered	....	At risk factors not considered
9. Appropriate action chosen for each problem	....	Inappropriate action chosen
10. Appropriate shared understanding of problems achieved	....	Shared understanding not achieved or inappropriate
11. Patient involved in management adequately and appropriately	....	Involvement in management inadequate or inappropriate
12. Appropriate use of time and resources in consultation	....	Inappropriate use of time and resources in consultation
13. Use of time and resources in long-term management appropriate	....	Inappropriate use of time and resources in long-term management
14. Helpful relationship with patient established or maintained	....	Unhelpful or deteriorating relationship with patient

SOURCE: From *The Consultation: An Approach to Learning and Teaching* (p. 67), by D. Pendleton, T. Schofield, P. Tate, and P. Havelock, 1984, Oxford, England: Oxford University Press. Reprinted with permission.

1986) and performance of tasks (Pendleton et al., 1984). Because Pendleton et al.'s tasks are so similar to components of patient-centered encounters outlined in this book, their Consultation Rating Scale is shown in full in Table 15.1.

Interviews With
the Patient and/or Physician

Interviews with the patient and physician might include some of the rating scales described above. As well, perceptions of patients and physicians about other aspects of the encounter central to the patient-centered approach can be assessed. Seminal research finding important associations with health assessed the agreement between doctor and patient and the degree of discussion of the symptom by using interviews with patients (Bass et al., 1986; Headache Study Group, 1986). Henbest and Stewart (1990) used such an interview to assess intermediate outcomes. An updated version of the questions used in these studies is shown in Table 15.2.

Combined Assessments

Three measures that illustrate the evolution during the past 20 years of measures of patient-centeredness and that lead to the tool presented later in this chapter are (a) Byrne and Long's (1976) checklist of behaviors with score values, which combines a count of doctor-centered and patient-centered statements of physicians with a weighting for patient-centeredness (Table 15.3); Brown, Stewart, McCracken, McWhinney, and Levenstein's (1986) scoring based on physicians' responses to patients' presentations (Table 15.4); and Henbest and Stewart's (1989) scoring based on degrees of responses of physicians to patient offers (Table 15.5).

Scoring Components 1, 2, and 3
of the Patient-Centered Approach

The most recent version of a scoring method of the patient-centered approach consists of three coding forms, one for each of the first three components: (a) understanding the disease and the illness experience (Table 15.6), understanding the whole person (Table 15.7), and finding common ground (Table 15.8).

(text continued on page 199)

TABLE 15.2 Interview With Patients

1.A. Would you say that your main problem(s) was discussed today?	1. completely 2. a lot 3. a little 4. not at all
B. Would you say that your doctor knows that this was one of your reasons for coming in today?	1. yes 2. probably 3. unsure 4. no
C. How well did the doctor understand the importance of your reason for coming in today?	1. very well 2. well 3. somewhat 4. not at all
D. How satisfied were you with the discussion of your problem?	1. very 2. satisfied 3. somewhat 4. not at all
E. What did the doctor say the problem was?	_____
F. Did you agree with his opinion?	1. completely 2. mostly 3. a little 4. not at all
G. How well understood did you feel by this doctor today?	1. very well 2. understood 3. somewhat 4. not at all
H. How much would you say that this doctor cares about you as a person?	1. very much 2. a fair amount 3. a little 4. not at all
I. Overall, do you feel the same, better, or worse after seeing the doctor today?	1. better 2. same 3. worse

SOURCE: Adapted from *A Study of the Patient-Centred Approach in Family Practice* (pp. 184-186), by R. J. Henbest (1985). Master's thesis, University of Western Ontario, London, Ontario, Canada. Adapted with permission.

TABLE 15.3 Byrne and Long's (1976) Checklist of Behaviors With Score Values

Doctor Centered Behaviour	Score Value	Incidence	I × SV
Offering self	1		
Relating to some previous experience	1½		
Direct question	1½		
Closed question	½		
Self-answering question (rhetorical)	½		
Placing events in time or sequence or place	2		
Correlational question	1½		
Clarifying	3		
Doubting	1½		
Chastising	1		
Justifying other agencies	1		
Criticising other agencies	1		
Challenging	2½		
Summarising to close off	1		
Repeating what patient said for affirmation	2		
Suggesting	1½		
Apologising	1½		
Misc. Prof. noises	1½		
Directing	1½		
Giving information of opinion	2		

Patient Centered Behaviour	Score Value	Incidence	I × SV
Giving or seeking recognition	1½		
Offering observation	3		
Broad question	2½		
Concealed question	3		
Encouraging	3		
Reflecting	4		
Exploring	2½		
Answering patient question	2		
Accepting patient ideas	4		
Using patient ideas	3		
Offering of feeling	2½		
Accepting feeling	4		
Using silence	4		
Summarising to open up	3		
Seeking patient ideas	4		
Reassuring	1		
Indicating understanding	2½		

Negative Behaviour	Score Value	Incidence	I × SV
Rejecting patient offers	−1		
Reinforcing self position (justifying self)	−1		
Denying patient	−1		
Refusing patient ideas	−1		
Evading patient questions	−1		
Refusing to respond to feeling	−1		
Not listening	−2		
Confused noise	−1		

TABLE 15.3 *(Continued)*

Doctor Centered Behaviour	Score Value	Incidence	I × SV
Relating to some previous experience	1½		
Directing	1½		
Clarifying	5½		
Doubting	3		
Chastising	2		
Justifying other agencies	1		
Criticising other agencies	1		
Challenging	4		
Summarising to close off	2		
Repeating what patient said for affirmation	3		
Giving information or opinion	3		
Advising	3½		
Terminating (direct)	1		
Suggesting	3		
Misc. Prof. noises	1		
Suggesting or accepting collaboration	4½		

Patient Centered Behaviour	Score Value	Incidence	I × SV
Offering observation	3½		
Broad question	3½		
Encouraging	5½		
Reflecting	6½		
Exploring	5½		
Answering patient question	4		
Accepting patient ideas	6		
Using patient ideas	4½		
Accepting feeling	5		
Using silence	7		
Summarising to open up	5½		
Seeking patient ideas	4½		
Reassuring	3		
Terminating (indirect)	4		
Indicating understanding	3		
Pre-directional probing	4½		

Negative Behaviour	Score Value	Incidence	I × SV
Rejecting patient offers	−1		
Reinforcing self position (justifying self)	−1		
Denying patient	−1		
Refusing patient ideas	−1		
Evading patient questions	−1		
Refusing to respond to feeling	−1		
Not listening	−2		
Confused noise	−1		

SOURCE: P. S. Byrne and B. E. L. Long (1976). *Doctors Talking to Patients* (pp. 162-163). London: Her Majesty's Stationery Office. Crown copyright is reproduced with the permission of the Controller of HMSO.

TABLE 15.4 Scoring Based on Physicians' Responses to Patients' Presentations

A	PATIENT BEHAVIOURS	
Expectations	Doctor *acknowledged*	Doctor *cut-off*
1.	Yes No	Yes No
2.	Yes No	Yes No
3.	Yes No	Yes No
4.	Yes No	Yes No
5.	Yes No	Yes No
6.	Yes No	Yes No
7.	Yes No	Yes No
8.	Yes No	Yes No
Feelings	Doctor *acknowledged*	Doctor *cut-off*
1.	Yes No	Yes No
2.	Yes No	Yes No
3.	Yes No	Yes No
4.	Yes No	Yes No
5.	Yes No	Yes No
6.	Yes No	Yes No
7.	Yes No	Yes No
8.	Yes No	Yes No
Fears	Doctor *acknowledged*	Doctor *cut-off*
1.	Yes No	Yes No
2.	Yes No	Yes No
3.	Yes No	Yes No
4.	Yes No	Yes No
5.	Yes No	Yes No
Prompts	Doctor *acknowledged*	Doctor *cut-off*
1.	Yes No	Yes No
2.	Yes No	Yes No
3.	Yes No	Yes No
4.	Yes No	Yes No
5.	Yes No	Yes No

B	PHYSICIAN FACILITATING BEHAVIOURS	
1.	9.	
2.	10.	
3.	11.	
4.	12.	
5.	13.	
6.	14.	
7.	15.	
8.		

SOURCE: From "Patient-Centered Clinical Method: Definition and Application," by J. B. Brown, M. A. Stewart, E. C. McCracken, I. R. McWhinney, and J. H. Levenstein, 1986, *Family Practice*, *3*, p. 79. Reprinted with permission.

TABLE 15.5 Scoring Based on Degrees of Responses of Physicians to Patient Offers

Practitioner _____		Purpose _____		
Scorer _____		Date _____		
Patient's offers		*Doctor's response(s)*		
(include: symptoms, thoughts, feelings expectations and prompts)	Ignore	Closed	Open	Specific facilitation (thoughts, feelings or expectations)
1. _____	0	1	2	3
2. _____	0	1	2	3
3. _____	0	1	2	3
4. _____	0	1	2	3
5. _____	0	1	2	3
6. _____	0	1	2	3
7. _____	0	1	2	3
8. _____	0	1	2	3
9. _____	0	1	2	3
10. _____	0	1	2	3
11. _____	0	1	2	3
12. _____	0	1	2	3
13. _____	0	1	2	3
14. _____	0	1	2	3
15. _____	0	1	2	3
No. of offers _____ Total score _____ Average score _____				
Signature _____				

SOURCE: From "Patient-Centredness in the Consultation: 1. Method for Measurement," by R. J. Henbest and M. Stewart, 1989, *Family Practice, 6*, p. 250. Reprinted with permission.

In general, after listening to the audio/videotape (either in segments or in full), the coder lists the patient and physician expressions under the appropriate headings for the first three components. For example, regarding Component 1, using a form such as the one shown in Table 15.6, the coder writes, in the patient's words: the patient's symptoms, prompts, ideas, expectations, feelings, and impact on function. Generally, after a second playing of the audio/videotape, the coder decides the appropriate categorization of the process for each symptom (or prompt, etc.) that had been written down. The process categories are preliminary exploration (yes/no), further exploration (yes/no), and cut-off (yes/no). Detailed definitions and examples can be found in Brown, Stewart, and Tessier (1994).

TABLE 15.6 Coding Form: Component 1—Understanding the Disease and Illness Experience

A. Symptoms	Preliminary Exploration	Further Exploration	Cut-off	SCORE	
*1. _____	Y N	Y N	Y N	___	
2. _____	Y N	Y N	Y N	___	
3. _____	Y N	Y N	Y N	___	
4. _____	Y N	Y N	Y N	___	
5. _____	Y N	Y N	Y N		
				**ST	☐

B. Prompts TT 6' OUTDENT	TT QC 6'	TT QC 6'	TT QC 6'	TT QC 6'	TT 6'
1. _____	Y N	Y N	Y N	___	
2. _____	Y N	Y N	Y N	___	
3. _____	Y N	Y N	Y N	___	
4. _____	Y N	Y N	Y N	___	
5. _____	Y N	Y N	Y N		
				ST	☐

C. Ideas					
1. _____	Y N	Y N	Y N	___	
2. _____	Y N	Y N	Y N	___	
3. _____	Y N	Y N	Y N	___	
4. _____	Y N	Y N	Y N	___	
5. _____	Y N	Y N	Y N		
				ST	☐

D. Expectations					
1. _____	Y N	Y N	Y N	___	
2. _____	Y N	Y N	Y N	___	
3. _____	Y N	Y N	Y N	___	
4. _____	Y N	Y N	Y N	___	
5. _____	Y N	Y N	Y N		
				ST	☐

E. Feelings					
1. _____	Y N	Y N	Y N	___	
2. _____	Y N	Y N	Y N	___	
3. _____	Y N	Y N	Y N	___	
4. _____	Y N	Y N	Y N	___	
5. _____	Y N	Y N	Y N		
				ST	☐

F. Impact on function					
1. _____	Y N	Y N	Y N	___	
2. _____	Y N	Y N	Y N	___	
3. _____	Y N	Y N	Y N	___	
4. _____	Y N	Y N	Y N	___	
5. _____	Y N	Y N	Y N		
				ST	☐

***GT ☐ + ☐ = ☐

NOTE: *Each quotation written down is called a statement.
          **Subtotal
          ***Grand total

TABLE 15.7 Coding Form: Component 2—Integrated Understanding of the Whole Person

Any statements relevant to FAMILY, LIFE CYCLE, SOCIAL SUPPORT, and PERSONALITY are listed below:

	Preliminary Exploration	Further Exploration	Cut-off	SCORE
*1. _____	Y N	Y N	Y N	_____
2. _____	Y N	Y N	Y N	_____
3. _____	Y N	Y N	Y N	_____
4. _____	Y N	Y N	Y N	_____
5. _____	Y N	Y N	Y N	_____
6. _____	Y N	Y N	Y N	_____
7. _____	Y N	Y N	Y N	_____
8. _____	Y N	Y N	Y N	_____
9. _____	Y N	Y N	Y N	_____
10. _____	Y N	Y N	Y N	_____
	GT [ ] + [ ] = [ ]			

NOTE: * Each quotation written down is called a statement.
** Grand total

Regarding Component 2, using the form shown in Table 15.7, the coder writes down any patient statements regarding family, life cycle issues, social support, personality, or other contextual issues in the patient's life. Next, the exploration of the issue is categorized as to whether preliminary exploration occurred, whether further exploration occurred, and whether discussion was cut off.

Regarding Component 3, two parts are used for ease of recording: doctor expressions and the interaction (Table 15.8). The coder lists under Part 1 the doctor's comments regarding problem definition and goals for treatment. Each comment then is categorized as to whether it was clearly expressed and whether an opportunity was provided for the patient to ask questions. On the bottom half of the form in Table 15.8, the same doctor comments are listed again, and any additional topics raised by the patient are listed as well. For each topic, the coder judges whether mutual discussion occurred and whether there is explicit clarification of agreement between the doctor and the patient. The coding forms allow scoring of each component and an overall score.

TABLE 15.8 Coding Form: Component 3—Finding Common Ground

Part 1. Doctor expressions	Clearly Expressed	Provided Opportunity to Ask Questions	SCORE
A. Problem definition			
1. _____	Y N	Y N	_____
2. _____	Y N	Y N	_____
3. _____	Y N	Y N	_____
4. _____	Y N	Y N	_____
5. _____	Y N	Y N	_____
			ST

B. Goals for treatment/management			
1. _____	Y N	Y N	_____
2. _____	Y N	Y N	_____
3. _____	Y N	Y N	_____
4. _____	Y N	Y N	_____
5. _____	Y N	Y N	_____
6. _____	Y N	Y N	_____
7. _____	Y N	Y N	_____
8. _____	Y N	Y N	_____
9. _____	Y N	Y N	_____
10. _____	Y N	Y N	_____
			ST

GT [＿＿] + 4 = [＿＿]

Part 2. The Interaction	Mutual Discussion	Clarification of Agreement	
A. Problem definition			
1. _____	Y N	Y N	_____
2. _____	Y N	Y N	_____
3. _____	Y N	Y N	_____
4. _____	Y N	Y N	_____
5. _____	Y N	Y N	_____
			ST

B. Goals for treatment/management			
1. _____	Y N	Y N	_____
2. _____	Y N	Y N	_____
3. _____	Y N	Y N	_____
4. _____	Y N	Y N	_____
5. _____	Y N	Y N	_____
6. _____	Y N	Y N	_____
7. _____	Y N	Y N	_____
8. _____	Y N	Y N	_____
9. _____	Y N	Y N	_____
10. _____	Y N	Y N	_____
			ST

Responded to disagreement with flexibility:

	Response	
1. _____	Y N n/a	_____
2. _____	Y N n/a	_____
		ST

GT [＿＿] + [＿＿] = [＿＿]

Summary

The reader has been presented with an overview of quantitative methods of assessing patient-centeredness for research or educational purposes. The most recent coding and scoring tool developed by the authors has been outlined in some detail.

16

Qualitative Approaches That Illuminate Patient-Centered Care

CAROL L. McWILLIAM

T he previous chapters focused on research methodologies of the scientific paradigm that use objective measures of process and outcome; this chapter illuminates the humanistic, interpretive methodologies of qualitative research. Just as Chapter 14 reviewed results of quantitative studies, this chapter presents key findings from the interpretive tradition.

Interpretive research methodologies elicit particulars about human nature and experience, extracting meaning and understanding from words, behaviors, actions, and practices of people (Zyzanski, McWhinney, Blake, Crabtree, & Miller, 1992). These methodologies aim to promote understanding of subjective, intuitive, dynamic, interrelated, context-dependent experiences of human life. The patient-doctor encounter constitutes one such experience.

Parallels between the patient-centered method and qualitative inquiry invite the application of this type of research to investigating patient-centered care. The patient-centered method is a process of acquiring understanding of a fellow human being. Patient-centered care focuses on the patient's disease and illness and on the patient as a whole person. In humanistic inquiry, the researcher and the research participant together strive to capture the needs, motives, and expectations of the participant to construct the interpretation of their experience. The patient-centered processes of finding common ground and building a relationship also have similarities to the process of humanistic inquiry. In both humanistic research methodologies and clinical practice of the patient-centered method, interpretive or hermeneutic analysis is a central component (Good, Herrera, Delvecchio-Good, & Cooper, 1985) of achieving the desired outcome, be it good research or good care.

Researchers have made limited use of humanistic inquiry for understanding the patient-doctor encounter. Therefore many opportunities to make a contribution through qualitative methodologies exist. McWhinney (1991) identified several areas of unfinished business to which researchers might specifically attend in the next 20 years. First, the task of making the implicit, or subconscious, rules of clinical methods explicit still must be accomplished. Second, important work is yet to be done in articulating the theory of medicine—in particular, the connections among human experience, life events, human relationships, and health and ill health. Third, the "high context" nature of patient-doctor communication requires research (Helman, 1991). Indeed, in all professional-patient communication, much is influenced by the hidden, invisible dimensions of "external" and "internal" context. Qualitative methodologies are essential for addressing these three areas.

This chapter provides an overview of qualitative approaches that respond to these opportunities for further research in patient-doctor communication. Examples illustrate: use of heuristic and action research approaches to make the implicit more explicit, thereby contributing to understanding that permits refinement of the practice of the patient-centered method; use of the grounded theory method to articulate and evolve the theoretical framework of the patient-centered approach; and use of phenomenology and critical theory research to enhance understanding of the high context of the patient-centered approach.

Making the Implicit Explicit

Much of the practice of the patient-centered approach to communication is premised on the art of medicine. This art is learned through practice by using intuitive personal knowledge and observation of role models who have mastered the art of patient-doctor communication. Thus one of the greatest challenges for researchers studying patient-doctor communication is making what is implicitly understood explicit, so that skillful approaches can be more consciously, and therefore more expediently, mastered. Practitioners as researchers may investigate their own experience, as shared by fellow professionals; or they may investigate the patient-centered approach as it is experienced by doctor and patients together; or they may focus on the patient's experience. Although many methodological options for qualitative investigation of the implicit exist, two approaches that illuminate the patient-doctor encounter particularly well are presented here: heuristic research and action research.

Heuristic research methodology is an approach in which the researcher engages in a personal inner search for deeper awareness of personal knowledge of some experience that he or she desires to understand better (Moustakas, 1981). The understanding discovered then is compared and contrasted with the understanding others have of similar experiences. The latter understanding is obtained through in-depth interview, participant observation, and/or comprehensive review of relevant literature. The approach requires a disciplined personal commitment to the process of searching for and studying meaning, for the self is always present (Moustakas, 1990) throughout a process of

> being open to significant dimensions of experience in which comprehension and compassion mingle; in which intellect, emotion, and spirit are integrated; in which intuition, spontaneity, and self-exploration are seen as components of unified experience; in which both discovery and creation are reflections of creative research into human ventures, human processes, and human experiences. (Moustakas, 1981, p. 216)

Miller (1992) engaged in a collaborative adaptation of heuristic inquiry to explore family physicians' experience of clinical encounters and the decision-making process used to manage these encounters on a daily basis. To make implicit practice explicit, Miller began by using in-depth interviews to acquire an understanding of how two experienced family physicians organized and managed their daily clinical encounters. Miller attended, in particular, to how experienced physicians anticipated "surprise" and "difficult" encounters and how they selected their patient-physician relationship style, including when to be family-oriented. On the basis of the understanding gained, Miller proceeded to explore the involvement of other key informants identified, including nurses. Data from all of these sources shaped further in-depth interviews with the original participants. Data elicited were combined with field notes of participant observation and with subsequent personal involvement as a self-reflective participant in the experience. A patient typology and taxonomy of descriptive terms for the encounters and their management gradually emerged.

Miller discovered four encounter types: (a) routine encounters for minor infections, trauma, reassurance, or examination; (b) dramas, which entailed complications, difficulties, or troubles associated with crises, bad news, family discord, or insoluble diagnoses; (c) transition ceremonies, which were "schedule busters" filled with such surprise challenges as presenting a new diagnosis of chronic disease; and (d) maintenance ceremonies, such as well-child or prenatal care visits or visits entailing management of chronic care needs.

Miller further discovered that classification of patients into these typologies normally was accomplished within the first 5 minutes of a visit and was based on the answers to several categories of questions: questions that (a) elicited the presenting concern, (b) determined why the patient was presenting at this moment in time, (c) determined what the patient wanted, (d) compared patient requests to the presenting concern, (e) assessed the physician's own gut feelings based on the total context of the patient-doctor relationship, and (f) assessed the patient's communication as being direct or indirect. Physicians in the study chose a contractual or mutual negotiation style for "routine" encounters, a shamanic style for "ceremonies," and an ever-changing style for "dramas."

Miller's typologies and decision-making strategies illuminate the physician's approach to a patient encounter in a way that facilitates efficient management of time and a patient-centered approach from the physician's perspective. These findings invite further qualitative investigation. For instance, researchers interested in the patient-centered method might frame their questions to ask: How do patients experience the clinical encounter? Do they perceive similar typologies? How do patients or patients and doctors together experience the management strategies that shape a clinical encounter? Do adoption of the typologies and implementation of the accompanying decision-making strategies alter the experience of the patient-centered method (e.g., does it mean that finding common ground is not an essential step in all encounters)? The answers to such additional questions would further illuminate the implicit practice of patient-centered care.

Understanding the process of patient-centered approaches can be derived also by using qualitative research approaches that capture the process as it unfolds. *Action research* methodology is one way of making the implicit processes explicit. Action research was developed by Kurt Lewin, a social psychologist, in the 1940s to create a bridge among theory, practice, and research. The central purpose of action research is to study processes through changing them and seeing the effect (Sanford, 1990). Thus the action researcher attempts to improve practical situations while developing or refining existing theory (Holter & Schwartz-Barcott, 1993; Lewin, 1951; McNiff, 1988; Nolan & Grant, 1993; Reason, 1988; Reay, 1986; Schon, 1987; Whyte, 1991).

In action research, the researcher involves research participants in assessing, planning, implementing, and evaluating action-oriented approaches to solving the everyday problems of concern. The basic steps of action research are those used to solve any practical problem or to learn any skill. By formalizing a research component as part of the everyday problem-solving process, researchers consciously obtain and document knowledge of the effect of everyday experiences. In this way, they create a concrete means of assessing intervention through conscious reflection on the experience. Rethinking past practice leads to theoretical reformulation of approaches, which, in turn, can lead to improved practice (McWilliam, 1992).

Two family physicians (Malterud, 1993; Seifert, 1992) have done trail-blazing work in patient-doctor communication by using action research methodology. Both worked with their own patients, engaging them as coresearchers, to discover ways of improving the process of care.

For example, in one study, Seifert (1992) and a group of his patients engaged in the process of finding common ground related to diagnostic labeling. Through collaborative participation, doctor and patients together developed a comprehensive list that purposefully eliminated terms the patients found difficult to define, difficult to understand, or difficult to accept because of their demeaning connotations. For several months, Seifert's action research team replaced several labels. For example, "schizophrenic" became the more understandable "reality disturbance"; "hypochondrias" became a less demeaning "sensitive person with physical response to stress"; and "psychopath" became "impulse control deficiency and ethical violation of own standards" (Seifert, 1992).

In subsequent evaluative focus group exploration, Seifert had participants address a number of questions related to partnership between physician and patient, negotiation methods, and continuity of care. Data reveal that patients experienced trust in response to the physician's providing listening and caring. Trust led to willingness, and willingness led to better participation in the health care process. The information exchange that then could transpire led to the acquisition of life management skills. Thus the process of patient-centered care led to empowering patients to take responsibility for and control of their own lives.

The invaluable dual outcome of using the action research approach is readily apparent. In the practice setting, Seifert and his colleagues improved the process of patient-centered care by jointly attending to it with patients. From a research perspective, Seifert gained explicit theoretical understanding of how the process of patient-centered care creates improved practice outcomes.

Articulating Theory

Patient-centered communication is an art; making the implicit explicit ultimately permits theory development. *Theory* is nothing more than explanation premised on observation, thought, and reasoning. Theories explain relationships between facts, occurrences, or other phenomena in nature. In the scientific paradigm, theories are formalized by testing hypotheses about the observed relationships (Little, Fowler, & Coulson, 1973). Formalized theories are valued as the basis of sound scientific practice. Because patient-centered care constitutes a critical component of medical practice, theory development in this area is important.

The first step in theory development is to discover the concepts, constructs, and patterns and relationships between concepts and constructs that relate to the phenomenon of interest. Because qualitative methodology aims to uncover the particulars of its subject matter and the patterns and relationships between and among these particulars, this type of inquiry readily lends itself to theory development. Although any qualitative methodology ultimately may contribute to theory development, one methodology is designed specifically to achieve this aim: the grounded theory method.

The *grounded theory* method of doing qualitative research is an approach to discovering, developing, and provisionally verifying theory through systematic collection and analysis of qualitative data pertaining to the topic under study. The researcher does not begin with a theory and then prove it. Rather, the researcher uses interviews, observation, or documents related to the actual experience of the area under study to identify common concepts and the relationships among them, thereby building concepts into constructs and constructs into an articulated theory that illuminates what is going on (Strauss & Corbin, 1990).

Researchers who use the grounded theory method hope to develop theories that ultimately will be related to others within the discipline. As well, grounded theorists aim to discover theories that will have useful applications to practice. Thus using grounded theory method holds the promise of developing the theory of the patient-centered method.

Taylor (1988) employed the grounded theory method to make explicit the implicit rules of initially informing patients that their diagnosis is breast cancer. Using constant comparative analysis (Glaser & Strauss, 1967) of transcriptions of interviews with 17 surgeons and participant observation accounts of 118 events in which the surgeons presented the diagnosis to patients, Taylor discovered four techniques of disclosing the bad news to patients: (a) candid, comprehensible communication, used in only 12 of the 118 events (10%); (b) admission of uncertainty, used in 18 of the 118 events (15%); (c) dissimulation, or the rendering of a diagnosis and prognosis, despite personal knowledge that neither could be medically substantiated, used in 35 (30%) of the 118 events; and (d) evasion, or failure to communicate a clinically substantiated prognosis, which occurred in 53 (45%) of the 118 events. Regardless of the technique used, three phases comprised the disclosure: preamble, confrontation, and diffusion of the bad news.

Taylor (1988) also found that the physicians imparting the bad news could be categorized as experimenters or as therapists. The experimenters ($n = 3$) fully disclosed the diagnosis, often providing more information than the patient sought, by using medical jargon and statistics to explain the prognosis. Experimenters relied on published studies to substantiate treatment recommendations, which were initiated quickly as part of the disclosure encounter. The encounter was staged in a sterile office with a desk between doctor and patient.

In contrast, the therapists ($n = 14$) were more patient-centered and relied on their own clinical acumen to guide the interview process. They offered less scientific information, used euphemisms to explain the diagnosis, and tended to assume the more traditional physician role—protecting patients from bad news and assuming full responsibility for any related decision making. Therapists tended to choose much more personalized offices outside the hospital as their setting for disclosure, frequently sitting on the same side of the desk as the patient, using the patient's first name, and divulging only information the patient might interpret as good news (e.g., "Your lump is in a good spot").

Taylor's (1988) grounded theory study findings illuminate how surgeons find ways to routinize the stressful task of telling bad news. Several insights have implications for those interested in the theory and practice of patient-centered communication. Findings illuminate the physician's power as the trustee of information and the challenge of obtaining a patient-centered balance between patients' rights and patients' interests in and abilities to contend with the information to be disclosed. Several questions that invite further qualitative inquiry to develop theory about the patient-centered method arise: How does a physician assess the patient's ideas, expectations, and feelings regarding disclosure of the diagnosis? How does the physician's understanding of the patient as a whole person interact with disclosure strategies and style? What role does finding common ground play in creating the nature of the disclosure process? How do doctors and patients experience the disclosure process as part of the overall relationship between them? What are the patient's perceptions of the importance of time and physical resources in the disclosure encounter?

Montgomery (1993) provides another excellent application of grounded theory method, which she used to explicitly illuminate communication of caring, long understood primarily at the intuitive level. Montgomery used participant observation and semistructured interviews of 45 health professionals to obtain an understanding of the nature and experience of caring communication from the perspective of caregivers. The *theory of caring* inductively derived describes caring communication as a way of being in relation to others. In Montgomery's theory, caring relationships encompass seven qualities: (a) a person orientation, rather than a role orientation, (b) concern for the human element in health care, (c) person-centered intention, (d) transcendence of judgment, (e) a hopeful orientation, (f) lack of ego involvement, and (g) expanded personal boundaries. Findings illuminate the patient-centered approach as being essential to communicating caring. Additionally, Montgomery's insights reveal that the intention to connect with, rather than to do to, a person can have a healing effect.

Montgomery's (1993) findings invite others to investigate further the value of the patient-centered method and to build theory specifically focused on this approach to caring. For instance, researchers might ask: How do patients experience patient-centeredness? How do doctors and patients together experience connectedness? How does patient-centeredness shape the experience of connectedness? How does connectedness shape the experience of illness and any healing that might subsequently transpire?

Capturing the Context

The patient-centered approach calls for an understanding of the whole person and his or her own unique experience of feeling unwell. Together, these concepts constitute the context of the patient's experience. *Context* is defined as "that which leads up to and follows and often specifies the meaning of a particular expression" and "the circumstances in which a particular event occurs" (Morris, 1982, p. 316). Thus study of the patient-centered method requires the application of research methodology that can capture the individual's context over space and time as he or she subjectively experiences it.

The patient-centered approach is a way of communicating, and communication is shaped by the context within which it occurs. Doctor and patient have both immediately and long ago internalized experience, expectations, and attitudes that shape how they individually and mutually enact and experience any encounter. This means that study of the patient-centered method would benefit from research methodology that captures the patient-doctor relationship in context.

Interpretive inquiry lends itself particularly well to capturing the context of communication. The focus of such research encompasses subjective experience, individual perceptions, shared language, interrelatedness, time and space considerations, and the context-dependency of human experience (Munhall & Oiler, 1986, p. 23). Two qualitative research methodologies are particularly helpful for studying the context of concern in the patient-centered approach: phenomenology and critical theory research.

Phenomenologists strive to articulate a coherent, cohesive description of existence, or of "being-in-the-world" (Swanson-Kauffman & Schonwald, 1988, p. 97). Understanding the research participant's personal experience necessitates active and extensive exploration of the participant's background, situation, and ongoing experiences. Experiences are interpreted in the context of time and space, with due consideration of historical, social, and physical dimensions of life. Meaning emerges out of the interactions between the individual and his or her world. All of the context and the individual's experience of it must be considered as together creating the experience as a whole (Hammond, Howarth, & Keat, 1991).

Phenomenological study of a patient's experience of illness can be used to both facilitate and demonstrate the effectiveness of the patient-centered approach. McWilliam, Brown, Carmichael, and Lehman (1994), for example, described how the individual's life context interacts with helping approaches used by professionals to shape patients' experiences of illness, and, in turn, their ability to manage following discharge from the hospital to home.

McWilliam et al. (1994) studied the discharge experiences of patients and their families and professional caregivers from the time they began in the hospital through 10 days postdischarge. Using participant observation, document review, and in-depth interviews of 21 patients and a chain sample of 22 family caregivers and 117 professionals involved in their care, McWilliam et al. discovered that, independent of the degree of severity of medical conditions and treatment protocols, patients' own mind-sets shaped their experience of discharge. *Mind-set* was defined as a way of thinking and feeling, reflecting purpose in life, intention, and will, and encompassing general attitude toward or perspective on life, attitude toward self and self-care, and attitude toward dependence on others. Patients' mind-sets interacted with maternalistic/paternalistic "doing to" and "doing for" approaches of family and professional caregivers.

Together, these factors created successful independence through the discharge experience or varying degrees of threatened independence and negatively perceived experience of discharge. Although these individuals often had more severe medical conditions for which they deferred to professional authority, patients with positive mind-sets managed to have successful discharge experiences, maintaining autonomy and a sense of control of their own care. Patients with more negative mind-sets forfeited independence to a degree that paralleled their negativity. Professionals and family caregivers responded to this negativity and helplessness with increased degrees of maternalism and paternalism, which, in turn, only made patients more lacking in self-confidence and self-esteem and more negative and helpless. Looking at this interaction in the context of a patient's entire life and health care experience allowed McWilliam et al. (1994) to uncover sources of patients' negativism, including unresolved grief, unanticipated role constraints, and lack of a sense of purpose in life.

Findings from this phenomenological study illuminate the importance of the patient's life and illness context and the potential of a patient-centered approach to care. Had this approach been used, underlying problems might have been addressed, and the patients' potential to experience success and independence following discharge might thereby have been enhanced. Beyond this, however, the research invites further exploration of context-related study of the patient-centered approach. Researchers have yet to explore these questions: How does a doctor come to understand a patient's life context as part of the immediate experience of disease and illness? How do patients experience life context as part of their present disease and illness? How do doctors and patients, interacting throughout the process of the patient-centered approach, cocreate the context of this disease and illness? How does the context created shape the experience of disease and illness?

Understanding of the larger sociocultural context in which patient-doctor communication occurs also might be explored. Critical theory methodology has particular applicability to this purpose. Waitzkin (1984) used critical theory methodology to make a contextual analysis of 30 tape-recorded medical encounters between doctors and patients. Interpretive analysis of entire interviews revealed how physicians unwittingly use professional status and authority to reinforce dominant social ideologies related to economic production, thereby subtly defining health as the capacity to work. In addition, Waitzkin found that the doctor controlled the patient's work life by determining the timing of returning to work, by exercising authority with regard to certification of fitness to work, and by medically managing leisure and pleasure. As well, endorsement of scientific medicine occurred, with the doctor turning socioemotional problems into a technical label (e.g., depression) objectively treated with polypharmacy, thereby mystifying the social roots of the patient's distress. Waitzkin concluded that despite the best intentions of well-motivated participants, medical encounters are embedded in social contexts that both shape and are shaped by the authority and status of the physician and scientific medicine. The microlevel processes of patient-doctor encounters tended to reinforce macrolevel patterns of domination and subordination in society.

Waitzin's (1984) research clearly illuminates a largely unexplored contextual dimension of patient-doctor communication and raises several research questions for those who would like to pursue study of the patient-centered method. For example, researchers might ask: How do patients experience the sociocultural context of the patient-doctor encounter? How would heightened sociopolitical understanding affect the doctor's application of the patient-centered method? How can doctors and patients work together to overcome the historically rooted sociopolitical characteristics of their relationship through patient-centered care?

Conclusion

Humanistic inquiry using interpretive qualitative research methodology permits particular achievements in the study of the patient-centered approach. Researchers may use these methodologies to make the implicit art of patient-centered communication more explicit. Theory development also may result. Additionally, qualitative methodologies permit exploration and understanding of the context-related components of patients' experiences, patient-doctor interactions, and patient-doctor relationships. Although a great diversity of methodologies exist, five examples that illuminate various aspects of the patient-centered approach were presented here. Practitioners and researchers alike are invited to rise to the challenge of the many additional research opportunities these studies suggest. Much more work is essential if we are to understand fully the nature and use of the patient-centered method.

17

Patient-Doctor Relationships Over Time

MOIRA STEWART

T he previous three chapters were reviews of quantitative and qualitative methods and findings. This chapter brings both qualitative and quantitative approaches to bear on a unique data set of interviews, permitting the study of patient-doctor relationships over time and, specifically, the description of patient-centeredness from one visit to the next.

The study arose out of an interest in one of the tenets of primary care and family medicine in Britain, Canada, and the United States: continuity of care. What do we know about the patient-doctor relationship in these settings of continuity? The studies reviewed in Chapters 14 to 16 used the snapshot approach, audiotaping or videotaping one sampled encounter and ignoring the fact that many visits preceded this one and that an opportunity exists for many more interactions following the study visit. In addition, most of the theoretical models on patient-doctor relationship imply the relationship is static and falls into one category or another. Some theoreticians, however, have recognized that different models might suit different circumstances (Szasz & Hollender, 1955).

Methods

The study sought to describe ongoing and evolving patient-doctor relationships by using part of a unique and rich data set of interviews between patients and doctors in community family practices in London, Ontario, Canada. These data were the audiotapes and subsequent transcripts of all visits of seven patients and their family doctors for 1 year. The patients were eligible if they were female, 25-80 years old, and new to the family doctor's practice. Three doctors—one male, two female—are represented in this data set, all with more than 2 years of experience in private practice. The seven patients had three to six visits during the year. When any eligible patient arrived at the doctor's office, the doctor asked permission to audiotape all visits for 1 year. The overall refusal rate was 47%.

Qualitative Analysis

The qualitative analysis had three goals:

1. To describe the evolving relationship between the doctor and the patient, with the ultimate goal of developing a typology of relationships
2. To identify turning points in the relationship (a *turning point* was defined as "a moment in the interaction that results in a change in the tone of the subsequent relationship")
3. To identify recurring themes in the relationships that might lead physicians and patients to better understand the process of developing a relationship

The qualitative analysis of the audiotaped visits proceeded in stages:

1. I listened to the audiotapes at the same time I proofread the transcripts, and after listening to *each visit*, I wrote comments on the important aspects of the visit. I tried not to restrict my observations to the patient-centered concepts I have been working with for the past 5 years.
2. I listened and read a second time, but now to the complete set of audiotapes and transcripts for each patient and his or her physician in the order they occurred during the year. After reading a whole year's set, I described or characterized the relationship.
3. I presented my observations and characterizations to Drs. William Miller and Benjamin Crabtree—one a family physician, the other an anthropologist at the University of Connecticut. They commented on the relationships and on my interpretations.

4. I summarized the transcripts (five pages down to one page), minimizing any interpretations, and I asked four colleagues—two academic family physicians, a nurse Ph.D., and a Ph.D. in social work—to read the summaries and to describe the relationships, identify any turning points, and identify themes arising from the sets of summaries. The purpose of these interpretations was to lend credibility to the results by guarding against any tendency on my part to see only what I wanted to see, "holistic fallacy," and to lend credibility by expanding the observations.

5. Working with my own interpretations and those of my six colleagues, I selected the descriptions and themes that were proposed by the majority, although the differing points of view and the vocabulary of the six will make an interesting future study of its own.

Findings:
Relationships Over Time

First, we could not identify clear turning points in the relationships from our analysis of the audiotapes and transcripts. Second, a very preliminary classification of types of patient-doctor relationships was suggested. In general, the relationships were organized into three types. The first type of relationship was described as *brisk, focused, trusting, straightforward,* and *unchanging.* This type of relationship was revealed in two patients. The doctor's role in these relationships was traditional, and although almost no discussion of emotions was observed, a bit of social chat and laughter did take place. The agreement among all of the interpreters was complete on the nature of these two relationships.

The second general type of relationships also included two patients. These relationships were described as *tolerant, warm, trusting, complex,* and *evolving but stable.* Both of these relationships were developed very early, one at the beginning of the first interview, and the second just toward the end of the first interview. In contrast with the first type of relationship, which was straightforward, this type was rich and complex.

The third type of relationship included three patients. These relationships, in general, were interpreted as *unfocused, inconsistent,* and *unstable;* however, the relationships were quite different from each other. One was a relationship fraught with uncertainty and tension at the beginning, evolving to a more supportive, trusting relationship in the middle, and ending on a cool but cooperative note after six visits. A second was described as inconsistent, spotty, wandering, business-like, and yet friendly at the same time. The last of these unfocused relationships was quite complex and interpreted differently by my colleagues. One said, for example, that the relationship was lacking in structure, and another suggested that an appropriate weaving back and forth occurred between the medical and psychosocial perspectives.

Two examples illustrate the evolving but stable type of relationship between patients and doctors. The first example, with Patient A, was characterized as a basically stable relationship. Nevertheless, this relationship evolved within the stability. The relationship moved from a beginning with *listening* and *caring*, through further *revelations* by the patient, to a third visit in which the patient *complimented* the doctor, and finally in the fourth visit, to evidence of a *partnership* between the doctor and the patient. The listening and caring portion of this relationship is illustrated by the following interaction:

Patient: That's quite a smile. Am I talking too much?
Doctor: No.

The patient then told long stories that were uninterrupted. The next phase of the relationship, labeled as "further revelations," is illustrated by this dialogue:

Patient: I'm feeling sort of nervous. I just needed that reassurance. Can I call between visits?
Doctor: Yes.

The patient then told a long story that she concluded by saying, "That's what's been happening to me." The doctor affirmed her by saying, "Thank you for telling me."

The third phase of this relationship is evident when the patient *complimented the physician*—"The best thing you did was recommend toast." And later, "I'm glad we cleared up about the medications; I was worried."

The final visit illustrates a fuller *partnership*, which is demonstrated by the following:

Patient: OK, that's the stomach. Have you any further comments?
Doctor: Sounds OK. [Laugh]

Later in the visit, the doctor asked the patient, "What do you think the pain is?"

The second relationship that indicated some evolution we also characterized as basically stable. This relationship, however, started with *many revelations* by the patient (Patient B) and *affirmation* by the physician and moved through a series of visits that included discussion about job and some *storytelling* but no deep revelations. Then the final visit was characterized predominantly by *social talk*. The depth in this relationship seemed to become less and less as time went on. In the first visit, the patient related a story about her teenage pregnancy and giving up the baby for adoption. The doctor replied, "That takes a lot of guts. Well, good for you." At the end of that visit, the patient brought up a concern: "I didn't think I'd ever come to a lady doctor." The doctor answered, "I know. My mother always took me to a male doctor, too, but a doctor is a doctor."

In the second and third visits, a discussion of job and family took place:

Patient: I got a job.
Doctor: Great.
Patient: My new job is linen services.
Doctor: Good for you.
Patient: I'm going to fitness now.
Doctor: Good for you.
Patient: My stepdaughter's now pregnant.
Doctor: It can happen to anyone.

The fourth and final visit of this relationship encompassed mostly social talk, some of which was repeated from the previous visit but forgotten by the doctor:

Patient: I'm working in linen services.
Doctor: Are you?
Patient: Didn't you know that? I didn't want to exercise anymore. It's got something to do with age.

Doctor: Don't talk to me about age.

Patient: I'll be thinking of you when I'm in Florida.

Two themes emerged from these data and deserve further comment. The first theme was *context* of the visit; it seemed to influence the evolution of the relationship. Five contextual factors influenced the seven relationships studied, and undoubtedly many others affect different patient-doctor relationships. The five revealed here are pregnancy, pressing clinical problem, pain, whether the patient was a health professional, and the physical examination. Other authors have written convincingly about the possibility of the social and clinical contexts of cases influencing doctors' decisions. The same physician may make a different decision under differing conditions or contexts (Christie & Hoffmaster, 1986).

The second theme revealed by the qualitative analysis was *continuity* of care. We are cautioned in the literature to be aware of costs, as well as benefits, of continuity of care. Some of the accepted benefits are the doctor's knowledge of the patient (McWhinney, 1975) and better patient compliance and satisfaction (Freeman, 1984, 1985). Arguments against personal continuity include patients becoming dependent on the doctor, and the physician relying too much on memory, rather than keeping written notes (Freeman, 1985).

None of the seven patients studied showed evidence of an unhealthy attachment or dependence. Rather, the deepening relationship and the mutual understanding experienced by Patient A seemed comfortable for the patient and doctor alike. In my view, this finding exemplifies the benefits of continuous personal relationships.

Patient B, however, described above, reveals to the doctor many problems at the first visit but reveals fewer and fewer problems as time goes on. She is perhaps an example of a second possibility in continuous relationships—namely, that of an evolution toward complacency and staleness.

Quantitative Analysis

The quantitative analysis, conducted after the above-mentioned qualitative findings, sought to shed light on two questions:

1. Is there a pattern of increasing or decreasing patient-centeredness over time?
2. Are any contextual factors (e.g., the kind of presenting problem) related to patient-centered scores?

With the small number of patients available, formal correlation analyses were not undertaken; rather, the patient-centered scores (derived using the method outlined in Chapter 15) were inspected for patterns.

Figure 17.1 shows the average scores over a number of visits: the total score, as well as scores for Components 1, 2, 3a, and 3b. The possible range for each score was 0-100. The average total score varied only slightly around the midrange of the scores (approximately 50), showing a slight rising trend. Scores for Component 1, understanding the illness experience, generally hovered around 40 and seemed to decrease somewhat until the fourth visit. Component 2, understanding the whole person, showed generally high scores in this sample, around 60-70, and rose somewhat until the fourth visit, when it fell. Component 3a, referring to that part of finding common ground concerning the clarity of the doctor's message and the opportunity for the patient to ask questions, scored relatively high in the 60-80 range, rising slightly in the later visits. Component 3b, the dimension of finding common ground concerning doctor and patient engaging in mutual discussion and finding agreement on a management plan, varied in scoring from visit to visit, ranging widely from 30-60.

Careful inspection of each patient's graph shows patterns that varied widely from patient to patient, and somewhat surprisingly, for four of the seven patients the scores varied markedly from visit to visit. The remaining three patients, however, demonstrated trends worthy of note.

The first exemplified scores on all components that were somewhat low on the first visit but that increased steadily during the four visits during the year (Figure 17.2). The largest increase was seen in the score for Component 3b, representing the degree to which the patient and doctor engage in mutual discussion and find agreement. We think this shows a doctor and patient learning to be patient-centered together.

The second example (Figure 17.3) illustrates two points: Although Component 2 generally was scored high, Component 1 was scored

(text continued on p. 226)

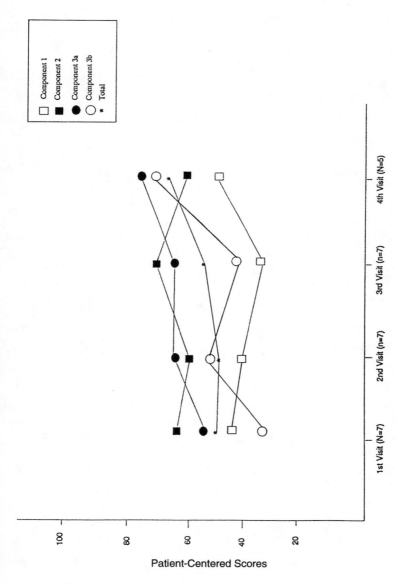

Figure 17.1. Average Scores for All Patients.

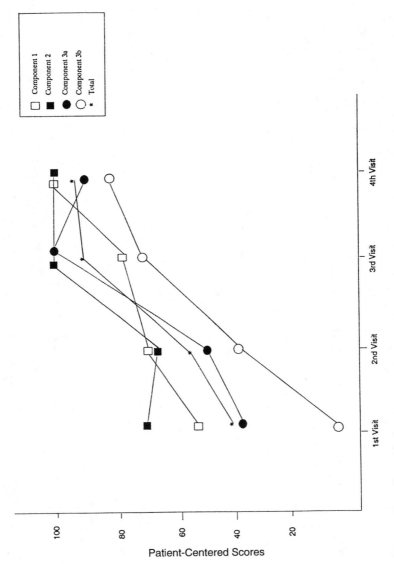

Figure 17.2. Example 1.

Patient-Centered Scores

□	Component 1		
■	Component 2		
●	Component 3a		
○	Component 3b		
*	Total		

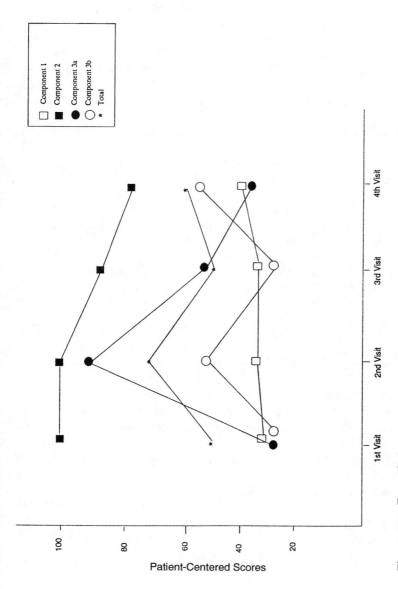

Figure 17.3. Example 2.

low, and a deterioration in scores from first visit to fourth visit occurred, particularly for Component 2 (understanding the whole person) and after the second visit, for Component 3a, as well. This doctor and patient, though working toward a relatively patient centered second visit, then began a tendency toward increasingly lower scores. This trend could be described as a slide after a strong start. One must look to patient and physician factors to help explain this finding because the context did not appear to vary from one visit to the next for this patient. It is possible for a patient to need to tell his or her story fully in the first few visits with a new doctor, and thereafter the need can diminish. Unfortunately, in this example, one senses that the doctor is distracted in the ability to listen and be present for this patient (Component 2), as well as in the ability to be clear about the proposed management plan (Component 3a).

The third example (Figure 17.4) shows a change in the focus of the visits at the third visit, the visit during which a pregnancy was diagnosed and the husband accompanied the patient. The scores on Component 2 (understanding the whole person) plummeted at the third visit. The scores on Component 3a (clarity of the physician's management plan and patient asking questions) were low at the third visit, when the husband was present, but rose at the fourth visit, when the husband was not present.

Two other pregnant patients (not shown in the figures) experienced low scores, supporting the conclusion that pregnancy care, with its regimens, impedes patient-centered care. Furthermore, one other patient, in addition to Example 3, was accompanied by another person, and she, too, experienced lower scores on that accompanied visit. It would appear that doctors have difficulty accomplishing their tasks in the presence of a third person. In Example 3, this appears to hold true to some degree for the straightforward task of Component 3a (doctor delivering a clear message and providing an opportunity for the patient to ask questions) but also, to a larger degree, for the more intimate task of understanding the whole person (Component 2).

The final point from this small-sample study is that the physicians who participated were not seen to display a consistent style (consistent patterns of scores on the components of patient-centeredness) from visit to visit or from patient to patient.

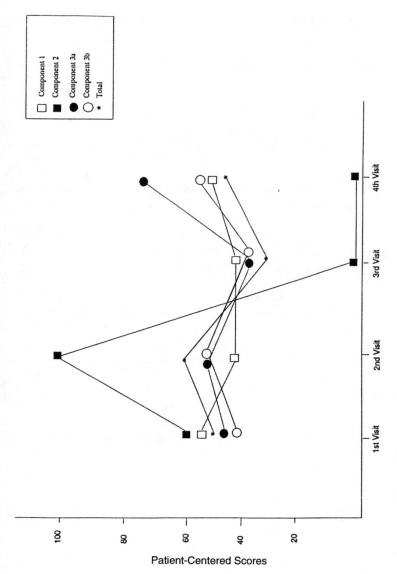

Figure 17.4. Example 3.

227

Conclusions

The qualitative study identified three evolving relationship types:

1. Focused, straightforward, unchanging
2. Complex, evolving, but stable
3. Markedly changing, with no discernable pattern over time

The context of the visit (whether for pregnancy or a physical examination) was found to change the evolving relationship.

The hypotheses derived from the qualitative study were tested and supported, although the majority of patients (4 of the 7) experienced communication that varied markedly from visit to visit. Less common were patterns of either increasing or decreasing patient-centeredness. The quantitative study revealed some evolution toward higher scores overall.

As well, two contextual factors were demonstrated to influence patient-centered scores, particularly on Component 2: the reason for the visit (pregnancy) and whether the patient was accompanied by another person.

The study leads us to ask questions about the nature of patient-centered care: To what extent is its genesis in the kind of physician or in the kind of problem the patient presents (e.g., pregnancy)? In what ways do the contextual factors, such as the nature of the patient's problem interacting with the guidelines for care of these problems (pregnancy care checklists), create a process that inhibits patient-centeredness? In what ways do some kinds of office situations, such as the patient being accompanied by another person, present barriers to patient-centered care? What disadvantages result when a doctor is patient-centered at some visits and not at others, especially with the same patient over time?

Conclusions

MOIRA STEWART

This book presents a clinical model and method relevant for all of medicine. No one medical specialty and no particular type of patient problem is better suited or less well suited to the approach outlined here. The patient-centered clinical method reveals the commonalities among medical disciplines, rather than their distinctions. Indeed, it is a clinical method that shares much with other health professions as well. All practitioners can acknowledge the importance of the six components of the patient-centered method: (a) exploring both the disease and the illness experience, (b) understanding the whole person, (c) finding common ground, (d) incorporating prevention and health promotion, (e) enhancing the relationship, and (f) being realistic.

One strength of the body of material contained in this book is that it represents a decade of work on four fronts simultaneously: (a) conceptual/theoretical development, (b) development of practical clinical approaches, (c) educational development, and (d) research.

Another strength of the patient-centered method is that it seeks to transcend some of the distinctions and limitations inherent in conventional medical models—specifically, the dichotomies between mind and body, art and science, thinking and feeling, the objective and subjective, and tacit and explicit knowledge.

The turning point that medicine is experiencing in its attempt to embrace wholes rather than parts (both the mind and the body, both the subjective and the objective) is one aspect of a larger societal transformation toward a postmodern era. This turning point is allied with other recent changes, such as the feminist movement, environmental action, and community development.

We have been struck by the fact that although the book presents the reader with a valuable, concise, diagrammatic framework that has been useful for teaching and that has stimulated excellent research ideas, there are limitations. The struggle to obtain clarity of vision for this book has resulted in two instructive diagrams: one on the patient-centered method and a parallel one on learner-centered teaching. The reader's eye follows lines dividing into two or three, focuses on neat boxes and overarching frames representing contextual components. None of these representations adequately depicts the complex interactive process that circles around and around while always moving. These somewhat linear diagrams, though extremely helpful for clinical practice, for teaching, and for clarity in research, do not succeed in representing the mysterious reality of a relationship between two people.

What does this book have to say to practicing clinicians? First, one must acknowledge that achieving patient-centered care is an important and somewhat daunting and long-term effort. It may be important also to say that aspiring to the practice of patient-centered medicine encompasses a *change of heart*, as well as a change of mind. The change implies a new order, one in which the patient is a partner in care. There is also a change in the way physicians see themselves. Finally, clinicians can be assured that patients are interested and will respond to being listened to, being respected, and working in partnership with doctors.

What conclusions can be drawn from this book for medical educators? One message rings through loud and clear: Learning the patient-centered approach is much more than skills training. To assist students in the all-important change of heart, attention must be paid to their stage of development and to opportunities for enhancing their self-awareness. Another key point for educators is the parallel process between the patient-centered model of clinical care and the learner-centered model of education. Finally, in our view, the next task should be to emphasize continuing medical education in order to assist practicing clinicians cope with the evolving demands of patients and the health care system.

What key messages does this book have for researchers? The research chapters attempt to model the important research thrusts required for further understanding of patient-centered care. Both qualitative and quantitative studies are required, particularly collaborative ones, to assess the benefits and to illuminate the processes of patient-centered care. Just as patient-centered concepts have translated into learner-centered guidelines for teachers, they also provide guideposts for researchers in their selection of methodology: The illness experience and patient-doctor relationship are suited to qualitative methodologies and the disease process and prevention are suited to quantitative methodologies.

Future Directions

As the practice of medicine evolves, some internal and external pressures will facilitate the adoption of patient-centered methods; others will impede patient-centered approaches. The future holds struggles to maintain and improve the level of clinical competence outlined in this book. We hope the progress that has been obvious in the past 5 years in undergraduate and residency programs can be enhanced by implementing the ideas presented in the education section of the book. We see a huge need for more development of continuing education for doctors who are already in practice and who live on a daily basis with the conflicts between patient-centered practice and other pressures on their time and commitment. The will to develop a more patient-centered approach needs to be allied with reflection on ways the clinical context may impede or enhance patient-centeredness.

We encourage medical theorists to improve on the schematic representations we have created to describe the patient-centered process of medical care. The flow of energy and information between patient and doctor as they work toward a shared goal over a period of weeks or months has been portrayed in this book in an admittedly oversimplified manner. The oversimplification, though extremely useful to the clinician and educator as a starting point, fails to capture the full richness and mystery of the human processes at work. We will join with others in meeting the challenge of creating ever more meaningful portrayals of patient-centered care.

Just as in clinical practice, the challenge in research on communication and the healing process will be to transcend the false dichotomy between objective and subjective knowledge. Although this book focuses on verbal behaviors, another whole field for the future is research on nonverbal aspects of communication.

Certain threads are woven throughout the chapters and sections of this book: sharing experiences, healing, connection, relationship, "walking-with," and partnership. The book reveals parallels between clinical medicine, advocating more emphasis on patient-centered clinical practice; teaching, advocating learner-centered education; and research, seeking to understand meaning and experience as well as disease.

One of the threads deserves special comment: *partnership.* The changes we imagine in medical care, education, and research are rooted in partnerships: between patients and doctors; between medical educators and medical students and residents; between continuing medical educators and practicing clinicians; among specialties within medicine; among the health professions; and among researchers of a variety of backgrounds, both quantitative and qualitative. Let us move medical care forward by first forging true and egalitarian partnerships in practice.

Appendix

Learning the Patient-Centered Method: Educational Objectives

OBJECTIVE	KNOWLEDGE	SKILLS	ATTITUDES
1. Exploring both the disease and the illness experience On the one hand, explores signs and symptoms of disease to develop a differential diagnosis; on the other hand, "steeps" oneself in the experience of patients to understand illness from their point of view.	Detailed knowledge of common diseases—especially their presentations and natural history. General knowledge of treatable life-threatening or disabling conditions even if rare—especially knowledge of early symptoms and signs. Understanding of why doctors and patients focus on organic manifestations of sickness and the limitations of this approach. Practical understanding of the distinction between disease and illness and the clinical relevance of this concept. Detailed knowledge of the common responses of persons to sickness—their ideas, expectations, feelings, and effects on function. Working knowledge of illness behavior and the sick role: why people go to doctors when they do and the benefits and responsibilities of being sick.	Facilitates communication by balancing the use of open-ended and closed-ended techniques. Avoids behavior that "cuts off" patients telling their own story of illness—for example, ignoring important cues, interruptions, excessive focus on disease, jargon, premature reassurance, reading the chart, closed posture. Elicits patients' experience of illness by facilitating discussion of their ideas, concerns, expectations, and the impact of illness on their lives. Pays attention to patients' feelings and responds appropriately to them. Searches for disease by zeroing in on cues to important disease processes. Conducts a reliable and efficient evaluation of patients' functional capacity—physical, emotional, and social. Recognizes early cues to impending disaster. Develops an efficient approach to the assessment of common presenting signs and symptoms. Performs a reliable and efficient physical examination of all body systems, in patients of all ages, in a manner that minimizes physical and emotional distress.	Willingness to become involved in the full range of difficulties that patients bring to their doctors, and not just their biomedical problems. Willingness to expend time, intellectual energy, and emotional energy in working with patients.

OBJECTIVE	KNOWLEDGE	SKILLS	ATTITUDES
1. Exploring both the disease and the illness experience (cont'd)		Avoids one-dimensional views of human sickness: skillfully weaves together the patient's story of illness with the physician's biomedical construct of the problem.	
		Critically analyzes data from any source—clinical evaluation, consultants' opinions, and the medical literature.	
		Deals with uncertainty and ambiguity appropriately by focusing on the needs and welfare of the patient, rather than on the physician's desire for precision. Recognizes when it is necessary to make decisions on incomplete or conflicting data.	
2. Understanding the whole person Understands patients' diseases and their experiences of illness in the context of their life settings and stages of personal development.	Deep knowledge of the human condition, especially the nature of suffering and the responses of persons to sickness. General understanding of the common effects of diseases on persons—physical, emotional, social, and spiritual. Practical knowledge of the common developmental issues of each stage of human development. Deep knowledge of the effects of serious illness of one member of a family on the rest of the family. Understands the characteristics and hazards of the caretaker role. Recognizes the impact of the family in ameliorating, aggravating, or even causing illness in its members. Knowledge of the cultural beliefs and attitudes of patients that might influence their care.	Applies the biopsychosocial model to define the appropriate contexts for understanding a patient's problems (e.g., molecules, tissues, organ systems, person, family, community). Defines patients' strengths. Interviews more than one family member at a time to gather information about the patient and about the influence of family interactions and relationships. Gathers information to construct a family genogram. Uses house calls to learn about the personal and family lives of patients. Takes an effective employment history to understand the role of work in causing or alleviating patient's problems. Addresses patients' spiritual values and explores, when appropriate, how patients come to terms with their suffering. Interviews patients within the context of their cultural background. Effectively interacts with patients, using an interpreter.	Respect for the fundamental worth of all persons. Even when patients do not comply with treatment or continue unhealthy lifestyles, the physician will demonstrate belief in their value as persons. Shows respect for the cultural values of all ethnic groups.

OBJECTIVE	KNOWLEDGE	SKILLS	ATTITUDES
3. Finding common ground Reaches a workable agreement with patients on the nature of their problems, appropriate goals of treatment, and roles of doctor and patient in management.	Deep knowledge of the scientific treatment of diseases commonly seen in practice. Understanding of the local folklore about common conditions seen. Awareness of the importance of patient autonomy. Understanding of issues that affect patient compliance. Understanding of how medical decision making is fundamentally a moral enterprise. Working knowledge of clinical epidemiology, especially regarding the predictive value of clinical and laboratory information and the critical appraisal of evidence.	Uses expertly the conventional methods of treatment for common problems (e.g., "watchful expectancy," modification of lifestyle, medications, office procedures, hospitalization, and referral). Also responds appropriately to emergencies and other serious problems, even if rare, for which early treatment makes a difference. Works with patients to manage effectively the full impact of disease and illness on themselves and their families. Collaborates with patients to empower them to take an active role in their own care. Determines patients' ideas about their problems, their preferences about treatment, and their concepts of the responsibilities of doctor and patient in management. Communicates information clearly to patients so that they are able to understand their problems and realize what may be done and what they can expect. Determines how much information regarding their condition patients want or are able to handle. Addresses differences of opinion with patients so that together they reach a conclusion that is both acceptable and safe for the patient. Knows when to give in gracefully to patients' urgent requests or demands and when, in the patients' best interests, it is essential to confront any differences of opinion.	Willingness to collaborate with patients about management, rather than needing always to "take charge." Awareness of personal values and cultural differences and how these might interfere with providing unbiased assistance to patients with different values or points of view.
4. Incorporating prevention and health promotion Practices a systematic approach to prevention and health promotion in the context of "ordinary" office visits.	Practical understanding of the importance of continuing comprehensive care and how this differs from episodic care.	Collaborates with the patient in developing a practical lifelong plan for health promotion and disease prevention.	Has enthusiastic interest in all three stages of prevention—primary, secondary, and tertiary.

OBJECTIVE	KNOWLEDGE	SKILLS	ATTITUDES
4. Incorporating prevention and health promotion (cont'd)	General awareness of the characteristics of effective screening tests.	At appropriate intervals, monitors patients regarding already recognized problems and screens for unrecognized disease on the basis of an individualized assessment of each patient's risks.	Invests time and energy to incorporate screening, prevention, and health promotion into day-to-day care of patients.
	Working knowledge of the evidence for or against the use of commonly recommended screening tests and the value of various preventive strategies (e.g., smoking counseling).	Uses the medical record system effectively as a reminder and also to document screening and prevention (e.g., problem lists, flow sheets, tickler files, computer systems).	Acknowledges the importance of health promotion activities.
	Ability to define a protocol for screening all patients in the practice for those conditions wherein screening has value.	Collaborates with the team to implement a program of screening and prevention in the practice.	
	Awareness of models of health promotion and their usefulness.	Enhances the patients' self-esteem and self-confidence in caring for themselves.	
5. Enhancing the patient-doctor relationship At every visit, strives to build an effective long-term relationship with each patient as a foundation for their work together and to use the relationship for its healing power.	Self-awareness of personal strengths and weaknesses in working with patients. Awareness of emotional reactions to patients.	Communicates effectively both verbally and nonverbally to connect with patients in meaningful and helpful ways.	Willingness to step into open-ended relationships with patients in which the demands are often unknown in advance.
	Understanding of the basic factors underlying an effective patient-doctor relationship—unconditional positive regard, empathy, and genuineness.	Creates a sense of security and comfort, both by his or her interactions with patients and by his or her very presence.	Risks exposing areas of weakness and vulnerability.
	Understanding of the healing power and spiritual aspects of the patient-doctor relationship.	Uses personal qualities effectively—empathy, generating trust and confidence, providing support and encouragement, being a model, and providing inspiration.	Risks being hurt.
	Working knowledge of the placebo effect.	Uses physical contact with patients to allay fears, to establish therapeutic bonds, and to provide comfort.	Has willingness to make personal sacrifices when necessary for the well-being of patients.
	Working knowledge of transference and countertransference.	Is able to "be with" patients in a healing relationship: attends fully to patients and their needs without always having to interpret or intervene.	Exhibits long-term commitment to the well-being of patients. The relationship is a form of covenant: Physicians promise to be faithful to their commitments even if patients do not comply or follow through on theirs.
			Willingness to "go to bat" for patients to protect them from the hazards of the health care system.

OBJECTIVE	KNOWLEDGE	SKILLS	ATTITUDES
5. Enhancing the patient-doctor relationship (cont'd)		Uses repeated contacts to build up personal knowledge of patients and their families. Helps patients deal with termination of the doctor-patient relationship by preparing them in advance and by providing opportunities to discuss their feelings about the relationship and about their loss. Recognizes which patients require special approaches to interviewing and treatment (e.g., recognizes patients who have unquenchable needs for support and, kindly but firmly, sets appropriate limits on the amount of time and energy he or she is able to expend).	
6. Being realistic Manages resources, especially time and energy, to provide optimal care for each patient in the context of the whole practice and the community in which the physician works.	Awareness of community resources. Understanding of the severe limitations of medicine to alter the natural course of disease. Understanding of the task of medicine: "To cure sometimes, to relieve often, to comfort always."	Organizes time effectively and efficiently and, as much as possible, stays on schedule. Recognizes when a patient's situation requires extra time even if this disrupts the schedule. Zeroes in on the heart of the problem: Does not lose the forest for the trees. Focuses on patients' prime needs but does not allow patients to ramble. Helps them identify their central concerns. Uses repeat visits effectively; does not try to do everything for every patient on each visit. Works effectively as a member of a health care team, contributing his or her expertise and delegating appropriately. Sets reasonable goals and priorities. Exhibits wise stewardship of limited community resources: balances needs of individual patients with the needs of the community. Avoids being overextended by limiting responsibilities to what realistically can be accomplished.	Has self-awareness of limitations and personal responses to stress. Accepts that physicians cannot be all things to all people. Able to say no without guilt. Expends time and energy building personal relationships within his or her family. Willingness to ask for help when needed.

References

Adjaye, N. (1981). Measles immunization: Some factors affecting nonacceptance of vaccine. *Public Health, 95,* 185-188.

Alonso, A. (1985). *The quiet profession: Supervisors of psychotherapy.* Toronto: Collier Macmillan Canada.

American College of Physicians. (1992). Guidelines for counselling postmenopausal women about preventive hormone therapy. *Annals of Internal Medicine, 117,* 1038-1041.

Anspach, R. R. (1988). Notes on the sociology of medical discourse: The language of case presentation. *Journal of Health Social Behaviour, 29,* 357-375.

Anstett, R. (1981). Teaching negotiating skills in the family medicine centre. *Journal of Family Practice, 12,* 503-506.

The aphorisms of Hippocrates. (1982). Birmingham, AL: Classics of Medicine Library.

Armstrong, D. (1977). The structure of medical education. *Medical Education, 11,* 244-248.

Archambault, R. D. (Ed.). (1974). *John Dewey on education: Selected writings.* Chicago: University of Chicago Press.

Audunsson, G. G. (1986). *Preventive infrastructure in family practice.* Reykjavik, Iceland: Iceland Ministry of Health.

Austen, Jane. (1981). *Emma.* New York: Bantam Classic Edition.

Bacon, Francis. (1973). *The advancement of learning.* New York: Rowman and Littlefield.

Baggs, J. C., & Schmitt, M. H. (1988). Collaboration between nurses and physicians. *Image: The Journal of Nursing Scholarship, 20*(3), 145-149.

Baker, S. S. (1985). *Information, decision making, and the relationship between client and health care professional in published personal narratives.* Ann Arbor, MI: University Microfilms International.

Baldwin, D. C. Jr., Daugherty, S. R., & Eckenfels, E. J. (1991). Student perceptions of mistreatment and harassment during medical school: A survey of ten United States schools. *Western Journal of Medicine, 155,* 140-145.

Bales, R. F. (1950). *Interaction process analysis: A method for the study of small groups.* Reading, MA: Addison-Wesley.

Balint, M. (1957). *The doctor, his patient, and the illness.* New York: International Universities Press.

Balint, M. (1964). *The doctor, his patient, and the illness* (2nd ed.). New York: International Universities Press.

Balint, M., Hunt, J., Joyce, D., Marinker, M., & Woodcock, J. (1970). *Treatment or diagnosis: A study of repeat prescriptions in general practice.* Philadelphia: J. B. Lippincott.

Bandura, A. (1986). *Social foundations of thought and action: A social cognitive theory.* Englewood Cliffs, NJ: Prentice Hall.

Barbee, R. A., & Feldman, S. E. (1970). A three-year longitudinal study of the medical interview and its relationship to student performance in clinical medicine. *Journal of Medical Education, 45,* 770-776.

Barfield, O. (1957). *Saving the appearances: A study in idolatry.* London: Faber & Faber.

Baskett, H. K., & Marsick, V. J. (1992). *Professional's ways of knowing: New findings on how to improve professional education* (New Directions for Adult and Continuing Education Series, No. 55). San Francisco: Jossey-Bass.

Bass, M. J., Buck, C., Turner, L., Dickie, G., Pratt, G., & Robinson, C. H. (1986). The physician's actions and the outcome of illness in family practice. *Journal of Family Practice, 23,* 43-47.

Battista, R. N., & Lawrence, R. S. (Eds.). (1988). Implementing preventive services. *American Journal of Preventive Medicine, 4*(Supp. 8).

Battle, C. U. (1975). Chronic physical disease. *Pediatric Clinics of North America, 22,* 525-533.

Becker, M. H., & Janz, N. K. (1990). Practicing health promotion: The doctor's dilemma. *Annals of Internal Medicine, 113*(6), 419-422.

Beisecker, A. E., & Beisecker, T. D. (1990). Patient information-seeking behaviours when communicating with doctors. *Medical Care, 28*(1), 19-28.

Belenky, M. F., Clinchy, B. M., Goldberger, N. R., & Tarule, J. M. (1986). *Women's ways of knowing: The development of self, voice, and mind.* New York: Basic Books.

Berger, J., & Mohr, J. (1967). *A fortunate man: The story of a country doctor.* New York: Pantheon.

Berquist, W. H., & Phillips, S. R. (1975). *A handbook for faculty development* (Vol. 1). Washington, DC: Council for the Advancement of Small Colleges, in Association with the College Center of the Finger Lakes.

Bertakis, K. D., & Callahan, E. J. (1992). A comparison of initial and established patient encounters using the Davis Observation Code. *Family Medicine, 24,* 307-311.

Bird, J., & Cohen-Cole, S. A. (1990). The three function model of the medical interview: An educational device. In M. S. Hale (Ed.), *Methods in teaching consultation-liaison psychiatry* (pp. 65-88). Basel, Switzerland: Karger.

Blacklock, S. M. (1977). Symptom of chest pain in family practice. *Journal of Family Practice, 4,* 429-433.

Blanchard, C. G., Ruckdeschel, J. C., Fletcher, B. A., & Blanchard, E. B. (1986). The impact of oncologists' behaviors on patient satisfaction with morning rounds. *Cancer, 58,* 387-393.

Borgman, A. (1992). *Crossing the postmodern divide.* Chicago: University of Chicago Press.

Bowen, M. (1976). Theory in the practice of psychotherapy. In P. J. Guerin (Ed.), *Family therapy: Theory and practice* (pp. 42-90). New York: Gardner.

Bowen, M. (1978). Toward the differentiation of self in one's family of origin. In M. Bowen (Ed.), *Family therapy in clinical practice* (pp. 529-547). New York: Jason Aronson.

Boyer, E. L. (1990). *Scholarship reconsidered: Priorities of the professorate.* Princeton, NJ: Carnegie Foundation for the Advancement of Teaching.

Brent, D. A. (1981). The residency as a developmental process. *Journal of Medical Education, 56,* 417-422.

British Medical Association. (1987). *The BMA guide to living with risk.* New York: Penguin.

Brock, C. D. (1986). Balint group leadership. *Family Medicine, 17,* 61-63.

Brod, M. I., & Hall, S. M. (1984). Joiners and nonjoiners in smoking treatment: A comparison of psychosocial variables. *Addictive Behaviour, 9,* 217-221.

Brody, H. (1992). *The healer's power.* New Haven, CT: Yale University Press.

Brookfield, S. B. (1985). *Self-directed learning: From theory to practice* (New Directions for Adult and Continuing Education Series, No. 25). San Francisco: Jossey-Bass.

Brookfield, S. B. (1986). *Understanding and facilitating adult learning: A comprehensive analysis of principles and effective practices.* San Francisco: Jossey-Bass.

Brown, J. B., Stewart, M. A., McCracken, E. C., McWhinney, I. R., & Levenstein, J. H. (1986). Patient-centered clinical method. Definition and application. *Family Practice, 3*(2), 75-79.

Brown, J. B., Stewart, M. A., & Tessier, S. (1994). *Assessing communication between patients and providers: A manual for scoring patient-centered communication* (CSFM Working Paper Series #94-1). London, Ontario: University of Western Ontario, Centre for Studies in Family Medicine.

Brown, J. B., Weston, W. W., & Stewart, M. A. (1989). Patient-centered interviewing: Part II. Finding common ground. *Canadian Family Physician, 35,* 153-157.

Broyard, A. (1992). *Intoxicated by my illness.* New York: Clarkson Potter.

Bruce, N., & Burnett, S. (1991). Prevention of lifestyle-related disease: General practitioners' views about their role, effectiveness, and resources. *Family Practice, 8*(4), 373-377.

Byrne, P. S., & Long, B. E. L. (1976). *Doctors talking to patients.* London, England: Her Majesty's Stationery Office.

Callahan, E. J., & Bertakis, K. D. (1991). Development and validation of the Davis Observation Code. *Family Medicine, 23,* 19-24.

Calnan, M. (1988). Examining the general practitioner's role in health education: A critical review. *Family Practice, 5*(3), 217-223.

Canadian Task Force on the Periodic Health Examination. (1979). The periodic health examination. *Canadian Medical Association Journal, 121,* 1194-1254.

Candib, K. (1988). Ways of knowing in family medicine: Contributions from a feminist perspective. *Family Medicine, 20*(2), 133-136.

Candib, L. M. (1985). The family approach at each moment. *Family Medicine, 17*(5), 201.

Candib, L. M. (1987). What doctors tell about themselves to patients: Implications for intimacy and reciprocity in the relationship. *Family Medicine, 19*(1), 23-30.

Candy, P. C. (1991). *Self-direction for lifelong learning: A comprehensive guide to theory and practice.* San Francisco: Jossey-Bass.

Cannon, W. B. (1900). The case method of teaching systematic medicine. *Boston Medical Surgical Journal, 142,* 31-36.

Carkhuff, R. R. (1987). *The art of helping VI.* Amherst, MA: Human Resource Development.

Carmichael, L. P. (1973). The family in medicine: Process or entity? *Journal of Family Practice, 3*(5), 562-563.

Carmichael, L. P. (1978). Introduction. In J. H. Medalie (Ed.), *Family medicine principles and applications* (pp. xv-xviii). Baltimore: Williams & Wilkins.

Carmichael, L. P., & Carmichael, J. S. (1981). The relational model in family practice. *Marriage & Family Review, 4*(1, 2), 123-133.

Carter, A. H. (1989). Metaphors in the physician-patient relationship. *Soundings, 72*(1), 153-164.

Carter, B., & McGoldrick, M. (Eds.). (1989). *The changing family life cycle: A framework for family therapy.* Boston: Allyn & Bacon.

Carter, H., & Jones, I. (1985). Measles immunization: Results of a local programme to increase vaccine uptake. *British Medical Journal, 290,* 1717-1719.

Carter, W. B., Belcher, D. W., & Inui, T. S. (1981, Winter). Implementing preventive care in clinical practice: II. Problems for managers, clinicians, and patients. *Medical Care Review,* pp. 195-216.

Casbergue, J. (1978). The role of faculty development in clinical education. In M. K. Morgan & D. M. Irby (Eds.), *Evaluating clinical competence in the health professions.* St. Louis: C. V. Mosby.

Cassell, E. J. (1985a). *The healer's art.* Cambridge: MIT Press.

Cassell, E. J. (1985b). *Talking with patients: II. Clinical technique.* Cambridge: MIT Press.

Cassell, E. J. (1991). *The nature of suffering and the goals of medicine.* New York: Oxford University Press.

Charon, R. (1986). To render the lives of patients. *Literature and Medicine, 5,* 58-74.

Charon, R. (1989). Doctor-patient/reader-writer: Learning to find the text. *Soundings, 72*(1), 137-152.

Cheren, M. (1983). Helping learners achieve greater self-direction. In R. M. Smith (Ed.), *Helping adults learn how to learn* (pp. 26-27). San Francisco: Jossey-Bass.

Cherry, J. D. (1984). The epidemiology of pertussis and pertussis immunization in the United Kingdom and the United States: A comparative study. *Current Problems in Pediatrics, 14,* 1-77.

Chickering, A. W. (1981). *The modern American college.* San Francisco: Jossey-Bass.

Christie, R. J., & Hoffmaster, C. B. (1986). *Ethical issues in family medicine.* New York: Oxford University Press.

Christie-Seely, J. (1984). *Working with the family in primary care.* New York: Praeger.

Cohen, S. J. (1985). An educational psychologist goes to medical school. In E. W. Eisner (Ed.), *The educational imagination: On the design and evaluation of school programs* (2nd ed., pp. 324-338). New York: Macmillan.

Cohen-Cole, S. (1991). *The medical interview: The three function approach.* St. Louis: Mosby/Yearbook.

Coleman, D. (1991, November 13). All too often, communicating is not a doctor's strong point. *The New York Times.*

College of Physicians and Surgeons of Ontario. (1988). *Annual report.* Ontario, Canada: Author.

Committee on Medical Care and Practice. (1982). *Medicine: The changing scene.* Toronto: Ontario Medical Association.

Cournoyer, B. (1991). *The social work skills workbook.* Belmont, CA: Wadsworth.

Cousins, N. (1979). *Anatomy of an illness as perceived by the patient.* New York: Norton.

Crookshank, F. G. (1926). The theory of diagnosis. *Lancet, 2,* 934-942, 995-999.

Crouch, M. (1986). Working with one's own family: Another path for professional development. *Family Medicine, 18,* 93-98.

Daloz, L. A. (1986). *Effective teaching and mentoring: Realizing the transformational power of adult learning experiences.* San Francisco: Jossey-Bass.

Davis-Barron, S. (1992). Cold hard death, cold hard doctors. *Canadian Medical Association Journal, 146*(4), 560-564.

de Leeuw, E. (1989). Concepts in health promotion: The notion of relativism. *Social Science and Medicine, 29*(11), 1281-1288.

Doherty, W. J., & Baird, M. A. (1986). Developmental levels in family-centered medical care. *Family Medicine, 18,* 153-156.

Doherty, W. J., & Baird, M. A. (1987). *Family-centered medical care: A clinical casebook.* New York: Guilford.

Donnelly, W. J. (1986). Medical language as symptom: Doctor talk in teaching hospitals. *Perspectives in Biology and Medicine, 30,* 81-94.

Donnelly, W. J. (1989). Righting the medical record: Transforming chronicle into story. *Soundings, 72*(1), 127-136.

Dostoyevsky, Fyodor. (1958). *The brothers Karamazov,* Vol. 1 (David Mayarshack, Trans.). London, UK: Penguin Books.

Doxiadis, S. (Ed.). (1987). *Ethical dilemmas in health promotion.* New York: John Wiley.

Dubos, R. (1980). *Man adapting.* New Haven, CT: Yale University Press.

Dubovsky, S. L. (1981). *Psychotherapeutics in primary care.* New York: Grune & Stratton.

Eagle, M. N. (1984). *Recent developments in psychoanalysis: A critical evaluation.* New York: McGraw-Hill.

Egbert, L. D., Battit, G. E., Welch, C. E., & Bartlett, M. K. (1964). Reduction of postoperative pain by encouragement and instruction of patients: A study of doctor-patient rapport. *New England Journal of Medicine, 270,* 825-827.

Eichna, L. (1980). Medical-school education, 1975-1979: A student's perspective. *New England Journal of Medicine, 303*(13), 727-734.

Eisner, E. W. (1985). *The educational imagination: On the design and evaluation of school programs* (2nd ed.). New York: Macmillan.

Ende, J. (1983). Feedback in clinical medical education. *Journal of the American Medical Association, 250*(6), 777-781.

Ende, J., Kazis, L., Ash, A., & Moskowitz, M. A. (1989). Measuring patients' desire for autonomy: Decision-making and information-seeking preferences among medical patients. *Journal of General Internal Medicine, 4*(1), 23-38.

Engel, G. L. (1977). The need for a new medical model: A challenge for biomedicine. *Science, 196,* 129-136. Copyright 1977 by the American Association for the Advancement of Science.

Engel, G. L. (1980). The clinical application of the biopsychosocial model. *American Journal of Psychiatry, 137*(5), 535-544.

Epp, J. (1986). *Achieving health for all: A framework for health promotion.* Ottawa: Health and Welfare Canada.

Epstein, R. M., Campbell, T. L., Cohen-Cole, S. A., McWhinney, I. R., & Smilkstein, G. (1993). Perspectives on patient-doctor communication. *Journal of Family Practice, 37*(4), 377-388.

Erikson, E. H. (1950). *Childhood and society.* New York: Norton.

Erikson, E. H. (1982). *The life cycle completed: A review.* New York: Norton.

Evans, B. J., Kiellerup, F. D., Stanley, R. O., Burrows, G. D., & Sweet, B. (1987). A communication skills programme for increasing patients' satisfaction with general practice consultations. *British Journal of Medical Psychology, 60,* 373-378.

Ewart, C. K., Taylor, C. B., Reese, L. B., & DeBusk, R. F. (1983). Effects of early postmyocardial infarction exercise testing on self-perception and subsequent physical activity. *American Journal of Cardiology, 51*(7), 1076-1080.

Faber, K. (1923). *Nosography in modern internal medicine.* (Jean Martin, Trans.). New York: Paul B. Hoeber.

Fabrega, H. (1978). *Disease and social behavior.* Cambridge, MA: MIT Press.

Fallowfield, L. J., Hall, A., Maguire, C. P., & Baum, M. (1990). Psychological outcomes of different treatment policies in women with early breast cancer outside a clinical trial. *British Medical Journal, 301,* 575-580.

Fields, H. J. (1990, March). About men: A whole new ball game. *New York Times Magazine.*

Fisher, L., Ransom, D. C., & Terry, H. E. (1993). The California Family Health Project: VII. Summary and integration of findings. *Family Process, 32*(1), 69-86.

Fisher, R., & Ury, W. (1983). *Getting to yes: Negotiating agreement without giving in.* New York: Penguin.

Forsyth, D. R., & McMillan, J. H. (1991). Practical proposals for motivating students. In R. J. Menges & M. D. Svinicki (Eds.), *College teaching: From theory to practice* (New Directions for Teaching and Learning Series, No. 45, pp. 53-65). San Francisco: Jossey-Bass.

Foss, L., & Rothenberg, K. (1987). *The second medical revolution—from biomedicine to infomedicine.* Boston: Shambhala.

Frank, A. (1991). *At the will of the body: Reflections on illness.* Boston: Houghton Mifflin.

Frank, S. (1991). Two green tomatoes: A case report regarding religion and health. *Family Systems Medicine, 9*(1), 69-75.

Frankel, R., & Beckman, H. (1989). Evaluating the patient's primary problem(s). In M. Stewart & D. Roter (Eds.), *Communicating with medical patients* (pp. 86-98). Newbury Park, CA: Sage.

Freeman, G. (1984). Continuity of care in general practice. *Family Practice, 11*(4), 245-252.

Freeman, G. (1985). Priority given by doctors to continuity of care. *Journal of the Royal College of General Practitioners, 35,* 423-426.

Freer, C. B. (1980). Self-care: A health diary study. *Medical Care, 18,* 853-861.

Frenette, J., & Blondeau, F. (1989). Balint groups in clinical training. In M. Stewart & D. Roter (Eds.), *Communicating with medical patients* (pp. 58-63). Newbury Park, CA: Sage.

Gagne, R. M. (1977). *The conditions of learning* (3rd ed.). New York: Holt, Rinehart & Winston.

Gagne, R. M., & Briggs, L. J. (1979). *Principles of instructional design* (2nd ed.). New York: Holt, Rinehart & Winston.

References 245

Galazka, S. S., & Eckert, J. K. (1986). Clinically applied anthropology: Concepts for the family physician. *Journal of Family Practice, 22,* 159-165.

Gerhardt, U. (1990). Qualitative research on chronic illness: The issue and the story. *Social Science and Medicine, 30*(11), 1149-1159.

Germain, C. B. (1984). *Social work practice in health care: An ecological perspective.* New York: Free Press.

Gilligan, C. (1982). *In a different voice: Psychological theory and women's development.* Cambridge, MA: Harvard University Press.

Gillis, A. J. (1993). Determinants of a health-promoting lifestyle: An integrative review. *Journal of Advanced Nursing, 18,* 345-353.

Glaser, B. G., & Strauss, A. L. (1967). *The discovery of grounded theory: Strategies for qualitative research.* Hawthorne, NY: Aldine.

Glasser, M., & Pelto, G. H. (1980). *The medical merry-go-round: A plea for reasonable medicine.* Pleasantville, NY: Redgrave.

Godkin, M. A., & Catlin, R. J. O. (1984). Office design. In R. E. Rakel & H. F. Conn (Eds.), *Textbook of family practice* (3rd ed.). Philadelphia: W. B. Saunders.

Goldberg, D. P., & Blackwell, B. (1970). Psychiatric illness in general practice; A detailed study using a new method of case identification. *British Medical Journal, 2,* 439-443.

Good, B. J., & Good, M. (1981). Meaning of symptoms: A cultural-hermeneutic model for clinical practice. In L. Eisenberg & A. Kleinman (Eds.), *Relevance of social science for medicine* (pp. 165-196). Boston: Reidel.

Good, B. J., Herrera, H., Delvecchio-Good, M., & Cooper, J. (1985). Reflexivity, counter-transference, and clinical ethnography: A case from a psychiatric cultural consultation clinic. In R. A. Hahn & A. D. Gaines (Eds.), *Physicians of Western medicine* (pp. 193-221). Boston: Reidel.

Greenfield, S., Kaplan, S., & Ware, J. E. (1985). Expanding patient involvement in care-effects on patient outcomes. *Annals of Internal Medicine, 102,* 520-528.

Greenfield, S., Kaplan, S. H., & Ware, J. E. Jr. (1988). Patients' participation in medical care: Effects on blood sugar and quality of life in diabetes. *Journal of General Internal Medicine, 3,* 448-457.

Haezen-Klemens, I., & Lapinska, E. (1984). Doctor-patient interaction, patients' health behaviour, and effects of treatment. *Social Science and Medicine, 19,* 9-18.

Hamilton, E., & Cairns, H. (Eds.). (1961). *The collected dialogues of Plato, including the letters.* New York: Bollingen Foundation.

Hammond, M., Howarth, J., & Keat, R. (1991). *Understanding phenomenology.* Oxford, UK: Basil Blackwell.

Hanckel, F. S. (1984). The problem of induction in clinical decision making. *Medical Decision Making, 4*(1), 59-68.

Haney, A. C. (1971). Psychosocial factors involved in medical decision making. In R. H. Coombs & C. E. Vincent (Eds.), *Psychosocial aspects of medical training.* Springfield, IL: Charles C Thomas.

Hartman, A., & Laird, J. (1983). *Family-centred social work practice.* New York: Free Press.

Haug, M., & Lavin, B. (1983). *Consumerism in medicine: Challenging physician authority.* Beverly Hills, CA: Sage.

Hawkins, A. H. (1986). A. R. Luria and the art of clinical biography. *Literature and Medicine, 5,* 1-15.

Hawkins, A. H. (1993). *Reconstructing illness: Studies in pathology.* West Lafayette, IN: Purdue University Press.

Headache Study Group of the University of Western Ontario. (1986). Predictors of outcome in headache patients presenting to family physicians: A one-year prospective study. *Headache, 26,* 285-294.

Heaton, C., & Kurtz, S. M. (1991). *Feedback forms.* Calgary, Alberta, Canada: University of Calgary.

Heaton, P. B. (1981). Negotiation as an integral part of the physician's clinical reasoning. *Journal of Family Practice, 6,* 845-848.

Helfer, R. E. (1970). An objective comparison of pediatric interviewing skills on freshman and senior medical students. *Pediatrics, 45,* 623.

Helman, C. G. (1991). Research in primary care: The qualitative approach. In P. G. Norton, M. Stewart, F. Tudiver, et al. (Eds.), *Primary care research: Traditional and innovative approaches* (pp. 105-124). Newbury Park, CA: Sage.

Helsing, K. J., & Szklo, M. (1981). Mortality after bereavement. *American Journal of Epidemiology, 114,* 41-52.

Henbest, R. J. (1985). *A study of the patient-centred approach in family practice.* Master's thesis, University of Western Ontario, London, Ontario, Canada.

Henbest, R. J., & Fehrsen, G. S. (1992). Patient-centredness: Is it applicable outside the West? Its measurement and effect on outcomes. *Family Practice, 9*(3), 311-317.

Henbest, R. J., & Stewart, M. (1989). Patient-centredness in the consultation: 1. Method for measurement. *Family Practice, 6,* 249-254.

Henbest, R. J., & Stewart, M. (1990). Patient-centredness in the consultation: 2. Does it really make a difference? *Family Practice, 7*(1), 28-33.

Hendley, B. (1978). Martin Buber on the teacher-student relationship: A critical appraisal. *Journal of Philosophy of Education, 12,* 144.

Hepworth, D. H., & Larsen, J. (1990). *Direct social work practice: Theory and skills* (3rd ed.). Belmont, CA: Wadsworth.

Hoffmaster, B. (1992). Values: The hidden agenda in preventive medicine. *Canadian Family Physician, 38,* 321-327.

Holter, I., & Schwartz-Barcott, D. (1993). Action research: What is it? How has it been used, and how can it be used in nursing? *Journal of Advanced Nursing, 18,* 298-304.

Huffman, M. C. (1993). Family physicians and the health care team. *Canadian Family Physician, 39,* 2165-2170.

Hulka, B. A., Kupper, L. L., Cassel, J. C., & Mayo, F. (1975). Doctor-patient communication and outcomes among diabetic patients. *Journal of Community Health, 1,* 15-27.

Hull, J. M. (1992). *Touching the rock of blindness.* New York: Random House.

Hummel, R. P. (1987). *The bureaucratic experience* (3rd ed.). New York: St. Martin's.

Hurowitz, J. C. (1993). Toward a social policy for health. *New England Journal of Medicine, 329*(2), 130-133.

Hurst, J. W. (1987). Foreword. In T. L. Schwenk & N. A. Whitman (Eds.), *The physician as teacher.* Baltimore: Williams and Wilkins.

Illich, I. (1976). *Medical nemesis: The expropriation of health.* New York: Pantheon.

Ingelfinger, F. J. (1980). On arrogance. *New England Journal of Medicine, 33*(206), 507-511.

Irby, D. M. (1978). Clinical teacher effectiveness in medicine. *Journal of Medical Education, 53,* 808-815.

James, William. (1958). *The varieties of religious experience: A study in human nature.* New York: The New American Library.

Jeffrey, R. W., Bjornson-Benson, W. M., Rosenthal, B. S., Lindquist, R. A., Kurth, C. L., & Johnson, S. L. (1984). Correlates of weight loss and its maintenance over two years of follow-up among middle-aged men. *Preventative Medicine, 13*(2), 155-168.

Jenkins, L. S. (1987). Self-efficacy: New perspectives in caring for patients recovering from myocardial infarction. *Professional Cardiovascular Nursing, 2*(1), 32-35.

Jerritt, W. A. (1981). Lethargy in general practice. *Practitioner, 225,* 731-737.

Johnson, J. E., Nail, L. M., Lauver, D., King, K. B., & Keys, H. (1988). Reducing the negative impact of radiation therapy on functional status. *Cancer, 61,* 46-51.

Jordan, J. V., Kaplan, A. G., Miller, J. B., Stiver, I. P., & Surrey, J. L. (1991). *Women's growth in connection: Writings from the Stone Center.* New York: Guilford.

Kaplan, R. M., Atkins, C. J., & Reinsch, S. (1984). Specific efficacy expectations mediate exercise compliance in patients with COPD. *Health Psychology, 3*(3), 223-242.

Kaplan, S. H., Greenfield, S., & Ware, J. E. (1989a). Assessing the effects of physician-patient interactions on the outcomes of chronic disease. *Medical Care, 275,* 5110-5127.

Kaplan, S. H., Greenfield, S., & Ware, J. E. (1989b). Impact of the doctor-patient relationship on outcomes of chronic disease. In M. Stewart & D. Roter (Eds.), *Communicating with medical patients* (pp. 228-245). Newbury Park, CA: Sage.

Kaprio, J., Koskenvou, M., & Rita, H. (1987). Mortality after bereavement: A prospective study of 95,647 widowed persons. *American Journal of Public Health, 77,* 283-287.

Katon, W., & Kleinman, A. (1981). Doctor-patient negotiation and other social science strategies in patient care. In L. Eisenberg & A. Kleinman (Eds.), *Relevance of social science for medicine* (pp. 253-279). Boston: Reidel.

Kestenbaum, V. (1982). *Humanity of the ill: Phenomenological perspectives.* Knoxville: University of Tennessee Press.

Klass, P. (1987). *A not entirely benign procedure: Four years as a medical student.* New York: G. P. Putman.

Klass, P. (1992). *Baby doctor.* New York: Random House.

Klaus, M. H., & Kennell, J. H. (1976). *Maternal-infant bonding.* St. Louis: C. V. Mosby.

Kleinman, A. (1988). *The illness narratives: Suffering, healing, and the human condition.* New York: Basic Books.

Kleinman, A. M., Eisenberg, L., & Good, B. (1978). Culture, illness, and care. *Annals of Internal Medicine, 88,* 251-258.

Klitzman, R. (1989). *A year-long night.* New York: Penguin.

Knowles, M. S. (1980). *The modern practice of adult learning: From pedagogy to andragogy* (2nd ed.). New York: Cambridge Books.

Knowles, M. S. (1984). *Andragogy in action: Applying modern principles of adult learning.* San Francisco: Jossey-Bass.

Knowles, M. S. (1986). *Using learning contracts.* San Francisco: Jossey-Bass.

Knowles, M. S. (1989). *The making of an adult educator: An autobiographical journey.* San Francisco: Jossey-Bass.

Kohut, H. (1971). *The analysis of the self.* New York: International Universities Press.

Kohut, H. (1977). *The restoration of the self.* New York: International Universities Press.

Konner, M. (1987). *Becoming a doctor: A journey of initiation in medical school.* New York: Viking-Penguin.

Koplan, J. P., Schoenbeum, S. C., Weinstein, M. C., & Fraser, D. W. (1979). Pertussis vaccine: An analysis of benefits, risks, and costs. *New England Journal of Medicine, 301*(17), 906-911.

Korsch, B. M., Gozzi, E., & Francis, V. (1968). Gaps in doctor-patient communication: I. Doctor-patient interaction and patient satisfaction. *Pediatrics, 42,* 855-871.

Kraan, H., Crijnen, A., Zuidweg, J., Vander Vleuten, C., & Imbos, T. (1989). Evaluating undergraduate training: A checklist for medical interviewing skills. In M. Stewart & D. Roter (Eds.), *Communicating with medical patients* (pp. 167-177). Newbury Park, CA: Sage.

Kraan, H. F., & Crijnen, A. A. M. (1987). *Maastricht History-Taking and Advice Checklist.* Amsterdam, Netherlands: Lundbeck.

LeBaron, C. (1981). *Gentle vengeance.* New York: Richard Marek.

Leder, D. (1990). Clinical interpretation: The hermeneutics of medicine. *Theoretical Medicine, 11,* 9-24.

Lee, J. (1993). Screening and informed consent. *New England Journal of Medicine, 328*(6), 438-439.

Lee, S. (1980). Interdisciplinary teaming in primary care: A process of evolution and resolution. *Social Work in Health Care, 5*(3), 237-244.

Leichtman, F. (1975). Social and psychological development of adolescents and the relationship to chronic illness. *Medical Clinics of North America, 59,* 13-19.

Levenstein, J. H. (1984). The patient-centred general practice consultation. *South Africa Family Practice, 5,* 276-282.

Levenstein, J. H., McCracken, E. C., McWhinney, I. R., Stewart, M. A., & Brown, J. B. (1986). The patient-centred clinical method: I. A model for the doctor-patient interaction in family medicine. *Family Practice, 3*(1), 24-30.

Levenstein, J. H., Brown, J. B., Weston, W. W., Stewart, M., McCracken, E. C., & McWhinney, I. (1989). Patient-centered clinical interviewing. In M. Stewart and D. Roter (Eds.), *Communicating with medical patients.* Newbury Park: Sage.

Levinson, D. J. (1978). *Seasons of a man's life.* New York: Knopf.

Lewin, K. (1951). *Field theory in social science.* New York: Harper.

Like, R., & Zyzanski, S. J. (1986). Patient requests in family practice: A focal point for clinical negotiations. *Family Practice, 3,* 216-228.

Little, M., & Midtling, J. E. (Eds.). (1989). *Becoming a family physician.* New York: Springer Verlag.

Little, W., Fowler, H. W., & Coulson, J. (1973). *The shorter Oxford English dictionary* (Vol. 2, 3rd ed.). Oxford, UK: Oxford University Press.

Longhurst, J. F., & Grant, H. F. (1989). Images of illness: Blindness. *Canadian Family Physician, 35,* 1623-1626.

Longhurst, M. F. (1989). Physician self-awareness: The neglected insight. In M. Stewart & D. Roter (Eds.), *Communicating with medical patients* (pp. 64-72). Newbury Park, CA: Sage.

Lowe, J. I., & Herranen, M. (1978). Conflict in teamwork: Understanding roles and relationships. *Social Work in Health Care, 3*(3), 323-330.

Lucas, A. F. (1990). Using psychological models to understand student motivation. *New Directions for Teaching and Learning, 42,* 103-114.

Mager, R. F. (1968). *Developing attitudes toward learning.* Palo Alto, CA: Fearon.

Mager, R. F. (1984). *Preparing instructional objectives* (rev. 2nd ed.). Belmont, CA: David S. Lake.

Maheun, B., Pineault, R., & Beland, F. (1987). Factors influencing physicians' orientation toward prevention. *American Journal of Preventative Medicine, 3,* 12-18.

Mailick, M. (1979). The impact of severe illness on the individual and family: An overview. *Social Work in Health Care, 5*(2), 117-128.

Malterud, K. (1993). The issue of validity regarding the contents of consultations. *Scandinavian Journal of Primary Health Care, 11*(2), 64-67.

Malterud, K. (1994). Key questions: A strategy for modifying clinical communication. *Scandinavian Journal of Primary Health Care, 12,* 121-127.

Maoz, B., Rabinbowitz, S., Herz, M., & Katz, H. E. (1992). *Doctors and their feelings: A pharmacology of medical caring.* New York: Praeger.

Marteau, T. M. (1990). Reducing the psychological costs. *British Medical Journal, 301,* 26-28.

Mattingly, C., & Fleming, M. H. (1994). *Clinical reasoning: Forms of inquiry in a therapeutic practice.* Philadelphia: F. A. Davis.

Mayeroff, M. (1972). *On caring.* New York: Harper & Row.

McCracken, E. C., Stewart, M. A., Brown, J. B., & McWhinney, I. R. (1983). Patient-centred care: The family practice model. *Canadian Family Physician, 29,* 2313-2316.

McCullough, L. B. (1989). The abstract character and transforming power of medical language. *Soundings, 72*(1), 111-125.

McDaniel, S., Campbell, T. L., & Seaburn, D. B. (1990). *Family-oriented primary care: A manual for medical providers.* New York: Springer Verlag.

McGinnis, J. M., & Hamburg, M. A. (1988). Opportunities for health promotion and disease prevention in the clinical setting. *Western Journal of Medicine, 149,* 468-474.

McIntyre, K. O., Lichtenstein, E., & Mermelstein, P. J. (1983). Self-efficacy and relapse in smoking cessation: A replication and extension. *Journal of Consulting and Clinical Psychology, 51,* 632-633.

McKeachie, W. J. (1978). *Teaching tips: A guidebook for the beginning college teacher* (7th ed.). Lexington, MA: D. C. Heath.

McNiff, J. (1988). *Action research principles and practice.* London: Macmilliam Education.

McPhee, S. J., Richard, R. J., & Solkowit, S. N. (1986). Performance of cancer screening in a university internal medicine practice. *Journal of General Internal Medicine, 1,* 275-278.

McPhee, S. J., & Schroeder, S. A. (1987). Promoting preventive care: Changing reimbursement is not enough. *American Journal of Public Health, 77,* 780-781.

McWhinney, I. R. (1972). Beyond diagnosis: An approach to the integration of behavioural science and clinical medicine. *New England Journal of Medicine, 287,* 384-387.

McWhinney, I. R. (1975). Continuity of care in family practice. *Journal of Family Practice, 2,* 373-374.

McWhinney, I. R. (1988). *Through clinical method to a more humane medicine in the task of medicine: Dialogue at Wickenberg.* Menlo Park, CA: Henry J. Kaiser Family Foundation.

McWhinney, I. R. (1989a, May). *An acquaintance with particulars.* Curtis Hames Lecture, presented at the Annual Spring Conference of the Society of Teachers of Family Medicine, Denver.

McWhinney, I. R. (1989b). The need for a transformed clinical method. In M. Stewart & D. Roter (Eds.), *Communicating with medical patients* (pp. 25-40). Newbury Park, CA: Sage.

McWhinney, I. R. (1989c). *A textbook of family medicine.* New York: Oxford University Press.

McWhinney, I. R. (1991). Primary care research in the next twenty years. In P. G. Norton, M. Stewart, F. Tudiver, et al. (Eds.), *Primary care research: Traditional and innovative approaches* (pp. 1-12). Newbury Park, CA: Sage.

McWilliam, C. L. (1992). Assessing interventions: Options for nurses in the primary care setting. In F. Tudiver, M. J. Bass, E. V. Dunn, et al. (Eds.), *Assessing interventions: Traditional and innovative methods* (pp. 208-218). Newbury Park, CA: Sage.

McWilliam, C. L. (1993). Health promotion: Strategies for the family physicians. *Canadian Family Physician, 39*, 1079-1085.

McWilliam, C. L., Brown, J. B., Carmichael, J., & Lehman, J. (1994). A new perspective on threatened autonomy in elderly patients: The disempowering process. *Social Science and Medicine, 38*(2), 327-338.

McWilliam, C. L., & Sangster, J. F. (1994). Managing patient discharge to home: The challenges of achieving quality of care. *International Journal for Quality Assurance in Health Care, 6*(2), 147-161.

McWilliam, C. L., & Wong, C. (1994). Keeping it secret: The costs and benefits of nursing hidden work in discharging patients. *Journal of Advanced Nursing, 19*, 152-163.

Medalie, J. H. (1978). *Family medicine principles and applications.* Baltimore: Williams & Wilkins.

Merriam, S. B. (1993). *An update on adult learning theory.* San Francisco: Jossey-Bass.

Merriam, S. B., & Caffarella, R. S. (1991). *Learning in adulthood.* San Francisco: Jossey-Bass.

Mezirow, J. (1991). *Transformative dimensions of adult learning.* San Francisco: Jossey-Bass.

Miller, G. E. (Ed.). (1961). *Teaching and learning in medical school.* Cambridge, MA: Harvard University Press.

Miller, W. L. (1992). Routine, ceremony, or drama: An exploratory field study of the primary care clinical encounter. *Journal of Family Practice, 34*(3), 289-296.

Miller, W. L. (1993). Physicians, patients, and third parties: Everybody's talking, but is anybody listening? [Editorial]. *Journal of Family Practice, 37*(4), 331-333.

Mishler, E. G. (1984). *Discourse of medicine: Dialectics of medical interviews.* Norwood, NJ: Ablex.

Mishne, J. M. (1993). *The evolution and application of clinical theory: Perspectives from four psychologies.* New York: Free Press.

Montgomery, C. L. (1993). *Healing through communication: The practice of caring.* Newbury Park, CA: Sage.

Morgan, M., Lakhani, A. D., Morris, R. W., & Vaile, M. S. (1987). Parents' attitudes to measles immunization. *Journal of the Royal College of General Practitioners, 37*, 25-27.

Morrell, D. C. (1972). Symptom interpretation in general practice. *Journal of the Royal College of General Practitioners, 22*, 297.

Morris, B. A. P. (1991). Case reports: Boon or bane? In P. G. Norton, M. Stewart, F. Tudiver, et al. (Eds.), *Primary care research: Traditional and innovative approaches* (pp. 97-104). Newbury Park, CA: Sage.

Morris, J., & Ingham, R. (1988). Choice of surgery for early breast cancer: Psychosocial considerations. *Social Science and Medicine, 27*, 1257-1262.

Morris, W. (Ed.). (1982). *American heritage dictionary* (2nd coll. ed.). Boston: Houghton Mifflin.

Moustakas, C. (1981). Heuristic research. In P. Reason & J. Rowan (Eds.), *Human inquiry: A sourcebook of new paradigm research* (pp. 207-217). New York: John Wiley.

Moustakas, C. (1990). *Heuristic research: Design, methodology, and applications.* Newbury Park, CA: Sage.

Mukand, J. (1990). *Vital lines: Contemporary fiction about medicine.* New York: St. Martin's.

Mundy, G. R. (1991). Presidential address of the SSCI: Can the triple threat survive biotech? *American Journal of Medical Science, 302*(1), 38-41.

Munhall, P. L., & Oiler, C. J. (1986). *Nursing research: A qualitative perspective.* New York: Appleton-Century-Crofts.

Munn, I. (1990). Poor communication main source of patient complaints in Maritimes registrar's report. *Canadian Medical Association Journal, 143,* 552-554.

Murray, T. (1991). Urgent need for MD's to relate better to patients. *Medical Post, 27* (42), 2.

National Research Council, Committee on Risk Perception and Communication. (1989). *Improving risk communication.* Washington, DC: National Academy Press.

Needleman, J. (1992). *The way of the physician* (pp. 132-133). London, UK: Arkana Penguin Books.

Newman, B., & Young, R. J. (1972). A model for teaching total person approach to patient problems. *Nursing Research, 21,* 264-269.

Nicki, R. M., Remington, R. E., & MacDonald, G. A. (1984). Self-efficacy, nicotine-fading/self-monitoring, and cigarette smoking behaviour. *Behavioral Research Therapy, 22,* 477-485.

Nolan, M., & Grant, G. (1993). Action research and quality of care: A mechanism for agreeing basic values as a precursor to change. *Journal of Advanced Nursing, 18,* 305-311.

Odegaard, C. E. (1986). *Dear doctor: A personal letter to a physician.* Menlo Park, CA: Henry J. Kaiser Family Foundation.

O'Hare, P., & Terry, M. (1988). *Discharge planning strategies for assuring continuity of care.* Rockville, MD: Aspen.

Orth, J. E., Stiles, W. B., Scherwitz, L., Hennrikus, D., & Vallbona, C. (1987). Patient exposition and provider explanation in routine interviews and hypertensive patients' blood pressure control. *Health Psychology, 6,* 29-42.

Payer, L. (1988). *Medicine and culture.* New York: Penguin.

Peabody, F. W. (1927). Care of the patient. *Journal of the American Medical Association, 88,* 877-882.

Pendleton, D., Schofield, T., Tate, P., & Havelock, P. (1984). *The consultation: An approach to learning and teaching.* Oxford, UK: Oxford University Press.

Perlman, H. H. (1979). *Relationship: The heart of helping people.* Chicago: University of Chicago Press.

Perry, W. G. Jr. (1970). *Forms of intellectual and ethical development in the college years.* New York: Holt, Rinehart & Winston.

Perry, W. G. Jr. (1981). *Cognitive and ethical growth: The making of meaning.* San Francisco: Jossey-Bass.

Pfeiffer, E. (1985). Some basic principles of working with older patients. *Journal of the American Geriatrics Society, 33,* 44.

Piaget, J. (1950). *The psychology of intelligence.* New York: Harcourt, Brace.

Pirsig, R. M. (1975). *Zen and the art of motorcycle maintenance.* New York: Bantam Books.

Pommerenke, F. A., & Dietrich, A. (1992). Improving and maintaining preventive services: Part 1. Applying the patient model. *Family Practice, 34*(1), 86-91.

Poulton, B. C., & West, M. A. (1993). Effective multidisciplinary teamwork in primary health care. *Journal of Advanced Nursing, 18*, 918-925.

Premi, J. (1991). An assessment of 15 years' experience in using videotape review in a family practice residency. *Academic Medicine, 66*, 56-57.

Preven, D. W., Kachur, E. K., Kupfer, R. B., & Waters, J. A. (1986). Interviewing skills of first-year medical students. *Journal of Medical Education, 61*, 842-844.

Putnam, S. M., Stiles, W. B., Jacob, M. C., & James, S. A. (1985). Patient exposition and physician explanation in initial medical interviews and outcomes of clinic visits. *Medical Care, 23*, 74-83.

Quill, T. E. (1983). Partnerships in patient care: A contractual approach. *Annals of Internal Medicine, 98*, 228-234.

Quill, T. E. (1989). Recognizing and adjusting to barriers in doctor-patient communication. *Annals of Internal Medicine, 111*, 51-57.

Rainey, L. C. (1985). Effects of preparatory patient education for radiation oncology patients. *Cancer, 56*, 1056-1061.

Ransom, D. C. (1993). The family in family medicine: Reflections on the first 25 years. *Family Systems Medicine, 11*, 25-29.

Ransom, D. C., & Vanderwoort, H. E. (1973). A significant group of intimates with a history and a future. *Journal of the American Medical Association, 225*, 1098-1102.

Reason, P. (1988). *Human inquiry in action: Developments in new paradigm research*. Beverly Hills, CA: Sage.

Reay, R. (1986). Bridging the gap: A model for integrating theory and practice. *British Journal of Social Work*, 16-64.

Reilly, P. (1987). *To do no harm: A journey through medical school*. Dover, MA: Auburn House.

Reiser, D., & Schroder, A. K. (1980). *Patient interviewing: The human dimension*. Baltimore: Williams & Wilkins.

Research Committee of the College of General Practitioners. (1958). Continuing observation and recording of morbidity. *Journal of the College of General Practitioners, 1*, 107.

Rogers, C. (1951). *Client-centered therapy: Its current practice implications and theory*. Cambridge, MA: Riverside.

Rogers, C. (1961). Significant learning. In C. Rogers (Ed.), *On becoming a person* (pp. 279-396). Boston: Houghton Mifflin.

Rolland, J. (1989). Chronic illness and the family life cycle. In B. Carter & M. McGoldrick (Eds.), *The changing family life cycle: A framework for family therapy* (pp. 433-456). Boston: Allyn & Bacon.

Rose, G. (1981). Strategy of prevention: Lessons from cardiovascular disease. *British Medical Journal, 282*, 1847.

Roter, D. L. (1977). Patient participation in patient-provider interaction: The effects of patient question-asking on the quality of interaction, satisfaction, and compliance. *Health Education Monographs, 5*, 281-315.

Roter, D. L., & Hall, J. A. (1991, November). *Improving psychosocial problem address in primary care: Is it possible, and what difference does it make?* Paper presented at the International Consensus Conference on Doctor-Patient Communication, Toronto.

Roter, D. L., & Hall, J. A. (1992). *Doctors talking with patients, patients talking with doctors*. Dover, MA: Auburn House.

Rudebeck, C. E. (1992). General practice and the dialogue of clinical practice. *Scandinavian Journal of Primary Health Care* (Suppl. 1), pp. 1-94.

Ruskin, J. (1981). *The stones of Venice* (abridged ed.). London: Bellow & Higdon.

Sackett, D. L., & Haynes, R. B. (1976). *Compliance with therapeutic regimens.* Baltimore: Johns Hopkins University Press.

Sacks, O. (1986). Clinical tales. *Literature and Medicine, 5,* 16-23.

Sanford, N. (1990). A model for action research. In P. Reason & J. Rowan (Eds.), *Human inquiry: A sourcebook of new paradigm research* (pp. 173-181). New York: John Wiley.

Sanson-Fisher, R., & Maguire, R. (1980). Should skills in communicating with patients be taught in medical schools? *Lancet, 2,* 523-526.

Savage, R., & Armstrong, D. (1990). Effect of a general practitioner's consulting style on patients' satisfaction: A controlled study. *British Medical Journal, 301,* 968-970.

Sawa, R. J. (1985). *Family dynamics for physicians: Guidelines to assessment and treatment?* Lewiston, NY: Edwin Mellen.

Schlesinger, E. G. (1985). *Health care social work practice.* Toronto: Times Mirror/Mosby.

Schoenbach, V. J., Wagner, E. H., & Karon, J. M. (1983). The use of epidemiologic data for personal risk assessment in health hazard/health risk appraisal programs. *Journal of Chronic Diseases, 36*(9), 625-638.

Schon, D. A. (1983). *The reflective practitioner: How professionals think in action.* New York: Basic Books.

Schon, D. A. (1987). *Educating the reflective practitioner.* San Francisco: Jossey-Bass.

Schwartz, M. A., & Wiggins, O. (1985). Science, humanism, and the nature of medical practice: A phenomenological view. *Perspectives in Biology and Medicine, 28*(3), 331-361.

Schwenk, T. L., & Whitman, N. A. (1987). *The physician as teacher.* Baltimore: Williams & Wilkins.

Seifert, M. H. Jr. (1992). Qualitative designs for assessing interventions in primary care: Examples from medical practice. In F. Tudiver, M. J. Bass, E. V. Dunn, et al. (Eds.), *Assessing interventions: Traditional and innovative methods* (pp. 89-95). Newbury Park, CA: Sage.

Sherwin, S. (1992). *No longer patient: Feminist ethics and health care.* Philadelphia: Temple University Press.

Siegler, M. (1985). The progression of medicine from physician paternalism to patient autonomy to bureaucratic parsimony. *Archives of Internal Medicine, 145*(4), 713.

Silver, H. K., & Glicken, A. D. (1990). Medical student abuse: Incidence, severity, and significance. *Journal of the American Medical Association, 263*(4), 527-532.

Smilkstein, G. (1978). The family APGAR: A proposal for a family function test and its use by physicians. *Journal of Family Practice, 17,* 1151.

Smilkstein, G. (1984). The physician and family function assessment. *Family Systems Medicine, 2,* 263-278.

Spiegel, D. A. (1981). Motivating the student in the psychiatry clerkship. *Journal of Medical Education, 56,* 573-600.

Stachtchenko, S., & Jenicek, M. (1990). Conceptual differences between prevention and health promotion: Research implications for community health programs. *Canadian Journal of Public Health, 81*(1), 53-59.

Starfield, B., Wray, C., Hess, K., Gross, R., Birk, P. S., & D'Lugoff, B. C. (1981). The influence of patient-practitioner agreement on outcome of care. *American Journal of Public Health, 71*(2), 127-131.

Stein, H. F. (1985a). *The psychodynamics of medical practice: Unconscious factors in patient care.* Berkeley: University of California Press.

Stein, H. F. (1985b). What is therapeutic in clinical relationships? *Family Medicine, 17* (5), 31.

Stephens, G. G. (1982). *The intellectual basis of family practice.* Tucson, AZ: Winter.

Stephens, G. G. (1993). Patients on patienthood: New voices from the high-tech area. *Journal of the American Board of Family Practice, 6*(2), 224-226.

Stetten, D. Jr. (1981). Coping with blindness. *New England Journal of Medicine, 305,* 458.

Stevens, J. (1974). Brief encounter. *Journal of the Royal College of General Practice, 24,* 5-22.

Stewart, M. A. (1984). What is a successful doctor-patient interview? A study of interactions and outcomes. *Social Science and Medicine, 19,* 167-175.

Stewart, M. A., Brown, J. B., & Weston, W. W. (1989). Patient-centred interviewing: Part III. Five provocative questions. *Canadian Family Physician, 35,* 159-161.

Stewart, M. A., & Buck, C. (1977). Physicians' knowledge of and response to patients' problems. *Medical Care, 15*(7), 578-585.

Stewart, M. A., McWhinney, I. R., & Buck, C. W. (1975). How illness presents: A study of patient behaviour. *Journal of Family Practice, 2*(6), 411-414.

Stewart, M. A., McWhinney, I. R., & Buck, C. W. (1979). The doctor-patient relationship and its effect upon outcome. *Journal of the Royal College of General Practitioners, 29,* 77-81.

Stewart, M. A., & Roter, D. (1989). *Communicating with medical patients.* Newbury Park, CA: Sage.

Stiles, W. B. (1986). Development of a taxonomy of verbal response modes. In L. Greenberg & W. Pinsof (Eds.), *The psychotherapeutic process: A research handbook* (pp. 161-199). New York: Guilford.

Stiles, W. B., & Putnam, S. M. (1989). Analysis of verbal and nonverbal behavior in doctor-patient encounters. In M. Stewart & D. Roter (Eds.), *Communicating with medical patients* (pp. 211-222). Newbury Park, CA: Sage.

Stiles, W. B., Putnam, S. M., Wolf, M. H., & James, S. A. (1979). Interaction exchange structure and patient satisfaction with medical interviews. *Medical Care, 17,* 667-681.

Stillman, P. (1977). Construct validation of the Arizona Clinical Interview Rating Scale. *Educational and Psychological Measurement, 37*(4), 1031-1038.

Strasser, T., Jeanneret, O., & Raymond, L. (1987). Ethical aspects of prevention trials. In S. Doxiadis (Ed.), *Ethical dilemmas in health promotion* (pp. 183-195). New York: John Wiley.

Strauss, A., & Corbin, J. (1990). *Basics of qualitative research: Grounded theory procedures and techniques.* Newbury Park, CA: Sage.

Styron, W. (1990). *Darkness visible.* New York: Random House.

Suchman, A. L., & Matthews, D. A. (1988). What makes the patient-doctor relationship therapeutic? Exploring the connexional dimension of medical care. *Annals of Internal Medicine, 108,* 125-130.

Swanson-Kauffman, K., & Schonwald, E. (1988). Phenomenology. In B. Sarter (Ed.), *Paths to knowledge: Innovative research methods for nursing.* New York: National League for Nursing.

Szasz, T. S., & Hollender, M. H. (1955). A contribution to the philosophy of medicine. *Archives of Internal Medicine, 113,* 585-592.

Szasz, T. S., & Hollender, M. H. (1956). The basic models of the doctor-patient relationship. *American Medical Association Archives of Internal Medicine, 97*, 585.

Tait, I. (1979). *The history and function of clinical records.* Unpublished M.D. dissertation, University of Cambridge, England.

Taylor, K. M. (1988). Telling bad news: Physicians and the disclosure of undesirable information. *Sociology of Health and Illness, 20*(2), 109-132.

Thomas, K. B. (1978). The consultation and the therapeutic illusion. *British Medical Journal, 1*, 1327-1328.

Thomas, K. B. (1987). General practice consultations: Is there any point in being positive? *British Medical Journal, 294*, 1200-1202.

Thompson, S. C., Nanni, C., & Schwankovsky, L. (1990). Patient-oriented interventions to improve communication in a medical office visit. *Health Psychology, 9*, 390-404.

Tiberius, R. G. (1986). Metaphors underlying the improvement of teaching and learning. *British Journal of Educational Technology, 2*(17), 144-156.

Toombs, K. (1992). *The meaning of illness: A phenomenological account of the different perspectives of physician and patient.* Norwell, MA: Kluwer.

Tough, A. (1979). *The adult's learning projects: A fresh approach to theory and practice in adult learning* (2nd ed.). Toronto: Ontario Institute for Studies in Education.

Toulmin, S. (1992). *Cosmopolis: The hidden agenda of modernity.* Chicago: University of Chicago Press.

Tresolini, C. P., & Shugars, D. A. (1994). An integrated health care model in medical education: Interviews with faculty and administrators. *Academic Medicine, 69*(3), 231-236.

Tuckett, D., Boulton, M., Olson, C., & Williams, A. (1985). *Meetings between experts: An approach to sharing ideas in medical consultations.* New York: Tavistock.

U.S. Preventive Services Task Force. (1989). *Guide to clinical preventive services: An assessment of the effectiveness of the 169 interventions.* Baltimore: Williams & Wilkins.

Veatch, R. (1972). Models for ethical medicine in a revolutionary age. *Hastings Center Report, 2*, 5.

Waitzkin, H. (1984). The micropolitics of medicine. *International Journal of Health Sciences, 14*(3), 339-380.

Wasson, J. H., Sox, H. C., & Sox, C. H. (1981). Diagnosis of abdominal pain in ambulatory male patients. *Medical Decision Making, 1*, 215-224.

Watson, J. (1984). *Health—A need for new direction: A task force on the allocation of health care resources.* Ottawa: Canadian Medical Association.

Watson, J. (1985). *Nursing: Human science and human care.* New York: Appleton-Century-Crofts.

Weed, L. L. (1969). *Medical records, medical education, and patient care.* Chicago: Year Book Medical Publishers.

Westberg, J., & Jason, H. (1991). *Providing effective feedback: A CIS guidebook for health professions teachers.* Boulder, CO: Johnson.

Weston, W. W., Brown, J. B., & Stewart, M. A. (1989). Patient-centred interviewing: Part I. Understanding patients' experiences. *Canadian Family Physician, 35*, 147-151.

White, K. L. (1988). *The task of medicine: Dialogue at Wickenburg.* Menlo Park, CA: Henry J. Kaiser Family Foundation.

Whitehead, A. N. (1975). *Science and the modern world.* San Francisco: Collins, Fontana.

Whyte, A., & Burton, I. (1982). Perception of risks in Canada. In I. Burton & R. McCullough, (Eds.), *Living with risk: Institute for environmental studies* (pp. 39-69). Toronto: University of Toronto.

Whyte, F. W. (1991). *Participatory action research*. Newbury Park, CA: Sage.

Wilde, O. (1915). *De Profundis, thirty first edition*. London: Methuen.

Wolfish, M. G., & McLean, J. A. (1974). Chronic illness in adolescents. *Pediatric Clinics of North America, 11*(21), 1043-1049.

Wood, M. L. (1991). Naming the illness: The power of words. *Family Medicine, 23*(7), 534-538.

Woods, M. E., & Hollis, F. (1990). *Casework: A psychosocial therapy*. New York: McGraw-Hill.

Wordsworth, W. (1988). *The prelude*. New York: Penguin.

World Health Organization (WHO), Regional Office for Europe. (1986a). *Health promotion: Concept and principles in action—A policy framework*. London: Author.

World Health Organization (WHO). (1986b). *Health promotion: A discussion document on the concept and principles* (ICP/HSR 602). New York: Author.

Wright, H. J., & MacAdam, D. B. (1979). *Clinical thinking and practice: Diagnosis and decision in patient care*. Edinburgh, Scotland: Churchill Livingstone.

Wulff, H. R., Pedersen, S. A., & Rosenberg, R. (1986). *Philosophy of medicine: An introduction*. Oxford, UK: Blackwell.

Zyzanski, S. J., McWhinney, I. R., Blake, R., Crabtree, B., & Miller, W. (1992). Qualitative research: Perspectives on the future. In B. Crabtree & W. Miller (Eds.), *Doing qualitative research: Research methods for primary care* (Vol. 3, pp. 231-248). Newbury Park, CA: Sage.

Index

About the Authors

Judith Belle Brown, Ph.D., is Assistant Professor in the Centre for Studies in Family Medicine, the Department of Family Medicine, at The University of Western Ontario, and in the Department of Social Work at King's College, London, Ontario, Canada. She conducts research in the areas of patient-doctor communication, physician well being, empowerment of the chronically ill elderly, the influence of culture on health, and woman abuse. She has published papers in *Social Science and Medicine; Family Practice: An International Journal; Canadian Medical Association Journal; Journal of Family Practice;* and *Family Practice Research Journal.* She is the coordinating author of a monthly column on patient-doctor communication in the *Ontario Medical Review,* and is known nationally for her workshops on the patient-centered method of practice. She earned her doctorate in Social Work from Smith College

Thomas R. Freeman, B.Sc., MClSc, M.D., C.C.F.P., began full-time academic practice in 1989 as an Assistant Professor of Family Medicine at The University of Western Ontario, and conducts a teaching

265

practice at the Byron Family Medical Centre of Victoria Hospital. He is a medical graduate of The University of Western Ontario, London, Ontario, Canada, and completed residency training in family medicine at Dalhousie University, Halifax, Nova Scotia, Canada. Before his current apppointment, he practiced medicine in Woodstock, Ontario, for 11 years, during which time he was involved with undergraduate medical education on a part-time basis. His areas of research interest include adverse effects to vaccines, risk perception and risk communication, and patient's use of metaphor. He has published in *Journal of Family Practice, Family Practice: An International Journal*, and *Canadian Medical Association Journal*.

Ian R. McWhinney, M.D., F.C.F.P., F.R.C.P, is Professor Emeritus in the Department of Family Medicine at The University of Western Ontario, London, Ontario, Canada. A native of England, he was educated at Cambridge University and St. Bartholomew's Hospital Medical School. For 14 years he was a General Practitioner in Stratford-on-Avon. In 1968, he was appointed Foundation Professor of Family Medicine at the University of Western Ontario, Canada, where he served until his retirement in 1992. He now has a postretirement appointment in the Centre for Studies in Family Medicine. His most recent book is *A Textbook of Family Medicine* (1989).

Carol L. McWilliam, M.Sc.N., Ed.D., is Assistant Professor in the Department of Family Medicine and the Faculty of Nursing at The University of Western Ontario, London, Ontario, Canada. She conducts research in the areas of health promotion and health services delivery, with a focus on professional-patient and interprofessional communication. She makes a unique contribution to the field as a qualitative research methodologist, with work published in *Social Science and Medicine, Family Medicine, Journal of Advanced Nursing*, and *International Journal of Quality in Health Care*.

Moira Stewart, Ph.D., is a Professor in the Department of Family Medicine and the Centre for Studies in Family Medicine at The University of Western Ontario, London, Ontario, Canada. She is an epidemiologist who, for the past 20 years, has done research on stress in relation to health and on communication between patients and doctors. She has published numerous articles in *Social Science and Medicine, Medical Care, Family Practice: An International Journal, Cana-*

dian *Medical Association Journal, Journal of the Royal College of General Practitioners,* and the *British Medical Journal.* She has been particularly active in fostering an international network of teachers and scientists of communication in medicine through the International Conference on Doctor-Patient Communication, the North American Primary Care Research Group's Interest Group on Doctor-Patient Communication. She has coedited a number of books, including *Communicating With Medical Patients* and *Tools for Primary Care Research.* She is an Honorary Member of the College of Family Physicians of Canada (1991) and received a Woman of Distinction Award for London, Ontario (1993).

W. Wayne Weston, M.D., C.C.F.P., F.C.F.P., is Professor of Family Medicine and Assistant Dean for Faculty Development in the Faculty of Medicine, The University of Western Ontario, London, Ontario, Canada. After graduating from the University of Toronto in 1964, he practiced in Tavistock, Ontario, for 10 years before joining the faculty at Western. He chairs the Ontario Network for Faculty Development of the Educating Future Physicians of Ontario Project. He has a special interest in medical education and the patient-doctor relationship and has published in such journals as *Canadian Family Physician, Canadian Medical Association Journal,* and *Academic Medicine.* He has led workshops for faculty on patient-centered interviewing, problem-based learning, and clinical teaching in Canada, New Zealand, and the United States. He received the Award for Excellence in University Teaching from The University of Western Ontario and the 3M Award for Excellence in Teaching in Canada.